SpringerBriefs in Modern Perspectives on Disability Research

Series Editors

Gabriel Bennett, Independent Researcher, Klemzig, Australia

Emma Goodall, Healthy Possibilities, Seaford, Australia

This book series on disability research is a comprehensive collection of research on disability and related issues. The series is designed to promote interdisciplinary collaboration and exchange, bringing together scholars and practitioners from different fields to share their perspectives and insights. Disability research is an interdisciplinary field that examines the social, cultural, historical, and political dimensions of disability. It encompasses a wide range of topics, including disability rights, accessibility, assistive technologies, healthcare, education, employment, and social welfare. Disability research scholars employ a range of theoretical and methodological approaches to understand the experiences of people with disabilities, as well as the ways in which disability intersects with other social identities such as race, gender, sexuality, and class.

The series seeks to advance knowledge and understanding of disability by publishing rigorous, innovative, and relevant research. It aims to promote disability rights and social justice by highlighting the ways in which people with disabilities are marginalized and discriminated against in society, and advocating for greater social inclusion and accessibility. The series also seeks to inform policy and practice by disseminating research findings that can help to shape policy decisions and contribute to positive social change.

Abdullah Al Shami · Abdulqadir J. Nashwan

Global Health and Disability

Challenges in Low- and Middle-Income
Countries

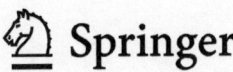

Abdullah Al Shami
AMC Therapy Pediatrics
Al Wakra Hospital
Hamad Medical Corporation
Doha, Qatar

Abdulqadir J. Nashwan🆔
Nursing & Midwifery Research
Department (NMRD)
Hamad Medical Corporation
Doha, Qatar

ISSN 3004-9709   ISSN 3004-9717 (electronic)
SpringerBriefs in Modern Perspectives on Disability Research
ISBN 978-981-96-4955-6   ISBN 978-981-96-4956-3 (eBook)
https://doi.org/10.1007/978-981-96-4956-3

This Springer imprint is published by the registered company Springer Nature Singapore Pte Ltd.
The registered company address is: 152 Beach Road, #21-01/04 Gateway East, Singapore 189721,
Singapore

If disposing of this product, please recycle the paper.

This book is dedicated to the millions of individuals with disabilities in low- and middle-income countries who continue to face barriers to inclusion, yet demonstrate remarkable resilience and strength every day. Your courage and determination inspire us to strive for a world where everyone, regardless of ability, has the opportunity to thrive.

We also dedicate this work to the families, caregivers, and advocates who tirelessly support individuals with disabilities, often in the face of immense challenges. Your love, dedication, and advocacy are the foundation upon which inclusive societies are built.

Finally, we dedicate this book to the next generation of leaders, researchers, and policymakers who will carry forward the mission of disability inclusion. May this work serve as a catalyst for your efforts to create a more just and equitable world.

Preface

Disability is a universal human experience, yet its impact is profoundly shaped by the socioeconomic and cultural contexts in which individuals live. In low- and middle-income countries (LMICs), the challenges faced by people with disabilities are often exacerbated by systemic barriers, limited resources, and deeply ingrained societal stigmas. Despite these challenges, there is a growing recognition of the need to address disability as a critical issue of global health, human rights, and sustainable development.

This book, *Global Health and Disability: Challenges in Low- and Middle-Income Countries*, seeks to shed light on the multifaceted challenges faced by individuals with disabilities in LMICs, while also exploring innovative solutions and strategies for fostering inclusion. Drawing on the latest research, international frameworks, and case studies, we aim to provide a comprehensive overview of the barriers to healthcare, education, employment, and social participation, as well as the policies and practices that can drive meaningful change.

Our motivation for writing this book stems from a shared belief in the importance of equity and inclusion. As healthcare professionals and researchers, we have witnessed firsthand the disparities faced by people with disabilities, particularly in resource-limited settings. This book is our contribution to the global dialogue on disability inclusion, with the hope that it will inspire action and collaboration among stakeholders across sectors.

We recognize that the journey toward disability inclusion is complex and ongoing. However, we firmly believe that by addressing the structural, cultural, and policy barriers outlined in this book, we can create a world where individuals with disabilities are empowered to live fulfilling and productive lives.

We invite readers to engage with the ideas presented in this book, to challenge existing norms, and to join us in advocating for a more inclusive and equitable future for all.

Doha, Qatar

Abdullah Al Shami PT, B.Sc.
Abdulqadir J. Nashwan RN, M.Sc., Ph.D.(c)

Acknowledgments

This book would not have been possible without the support, guidance, and contributions of numerous individuals and organizations. We are deeply grateful to all those who have played a role in bringing this project to fruition.

First and foremost, we would like to express our heartfelt gratitude to Hamad Medical Corporation and Qatar University for their unwavering support and encouragement throughout this journey. Their commitment to advancing global health and disability research has been instrumental in shaping this work.

We extend our sincere thanks to our colleagues and peers who provided valuable insights, feedback, and expertise during the development of this book. Special thanks to the World Health Organization (WHO), United Nations Children's Fund (UNICEF), and the World Bank for their groundbreaking research and reports, which served as foundational resources for our discussions.

We are also indebted to the countless individuals with disabilities, their families, and communities in low- and middle-income countries (LMICs) who shared their experiences and challenges. Their resilience and strength inspired us to delve deeper into the issues of disability inclusion and advocate for meaningful change.

To our editors, reviewers, and publishers, we thank you for your patience, meticulous attention to detail, and commitment to ensuring the quality of this book. Your efforts have been invaluable in bringing this project to life.

Finally, we would like to acknowledge the support of our families and friends, who have been a constant source of encouragement and motivation. Your belief in our work has been a driving force behind this endeavor.

This book is a collective effort, and we are deeply grateful to everyone who contributed to its creation. We hope it serves as a meaningful resource for researchers, policymakers, and advocates working toward a more inclusive and equitable world.

Contents

1 **Introduction to Disability in Low- and Middle-Income Countries**   1
   1.1   Definitions of Disability (WHO, CRPD)   1
   1.2   Global and Regional Prevalence   3
         1.2.1   Global Prevalence   3
         1.2.2   Disability in Low- and Middle-Income Countries
                 (LMICs)   4
         1.2.3   Regional Prevalence of Disability in LMICs   4
         1.2.4   Comparative Analysis of Disability Prevalence
                 in Children   5
         1.2.5   Healthcare Access   5
         1.2.6   Stigma and Social Exclusion   6
         1.2.7   Poverty and Disability   6
   1.3   Types of Disabilities in LMICs   7
         1.3.1   Physical Disabilities   7
         1.3.2   Visual and Hearing Impairments   7
         1.3.3   Intellectual Disabilities   8
         1.3.4   Mental Health Disorders   8
   1.4   Compounding Factors   8
   1.5   The Importance of Addressing Disability in LMICs   9
   1.6   Conclusion   10
   References   10

2 **Healthcare Access for People with Disabilities in LMICs**   13
   2.1   The Prevalence and Impact of Disability in LMICs   13
   2.2   Key Barriers to Healthcare Access   14
         2.2.1   Economic Barriers   14
         2.2.2   Physical and Infrastructure Barriers   15
         2.2.3   Social and Cultural Barriers   15

    2.3   Frameworks for Understanding Healthcare Access Barriers   16
           2.3.1   The Social Model of Disability   16
           2.3.2   The Capability Approach   16
    2.4   The Role of International Policy in Improving Healthcare Access ...   17
    2.5   Strategies for Enhancing Healthcare Access for People
           with Disabilities in Low- and Middle-Income Countries   17
           2.5.1   Policy Development and Advocacy   18
           2.5.2   Improving Healthcare Infrastructure   18
           2.5.3   Education and Training for Healthcare Providers   19
    2.6   Conclusion   19
    References   19

3   Educational Inclusion for People with Disabilities in LMICs   23
    3.1   Context of Educational Inclusion in LMICs   23
    3.2   Barriers to Education for People with Disabilities in LMICs   24
    3.3   Effectiveness of Inclusive Education Policies   27
    3.4   Outcomes of Educational Interventions   28
    3.5   Gaps in Research   28
    3.6   Recommendations for Future Studies   30
    3.7   Conclusion   30
    References   31

4   Employment and Disability in LMICs   33
    4.1   Barriers to Employment   33
    4.2   Facilitators of Employment   35
    4.3   Economic Implications   36
    4.4   Research Gaps and Recommendations   38
    4.5   Conclusion   39
    References   39

5   Socio-Cultural Perceptions of Disability in LMICs   41
    5.1   Understanding Cultural Beliefs and Norms   41
    5.2   Religious Influences on Disability Perception   42
    5.3   Stigma and Discrimination   42
    5.4   Policy and Advocacy: Addressing Socio-Cultural Barriers   43
    5.5   Case Studies and Best Practices   43
    5.6   Future Directions   44
    5.7   Conclusion   44
    References   45

6   Disability Rights and Policy in LMICs 47
    6.1   Overview 47
    6.2   International Conventions and Frameworks 48
    6.3   National Legal Frameworks in LMICs 48
    6.4   Barriers to Implementation of Disability Rights 49
    6.5   The Role of Advocacy Groups and Disabled People's
          Organizations (DPOs) 49
    6.6   Advancing Disability Rights: Effective Policies and Approaches ... 50
    6.7   Policy Gaps and Future Directions 50
    6.8   Conclusion 51
    References 51

**7   Innovations and Future Directions in Disability Research
    and Practice** 53
    7.1   Overview 53
    7.2   Technological Advancements 53
         7.2.1   Assistive Technologies 53
         7.2.2   Digital Innovations 54
         7.2.3   Data-Driven Inclusion 55
         7.2.4   Social Inclusion Interventions in LMICs 55
    7.3   Access to Rehabilitation Services in LMICs 56
    7.4   Community Support for Persons with Disabilities 57
    7.5   Innovative Care Models 57
         7.5.1   Community-Based Rehabilitation (CBR) 57
         7.5.2   Family-Centered Care (FCC) 58
         7.5.3   Inclusive Education 58
    7.6   Policy Interventions 58
         7.6.1   Legal Frameworks 58
         7.6.2   Multisectoral Collaboration 58
         7.6.3   Financial Incentives 59
    7.7   Research Agenda 59
    7.8   Conclusion 59
    References 60

Chapter 1
Introduction to Disability in Low- and Middle-Income Countries

Abstract This chapter explores the intersection of disability and socioeconomic development in low- and middle-income countries (LMICs), emphasizing its implications for global health and equity. It begins with a comprehensive definition of disability informed by the World Health Organization (WHO) and the Convention on the Rights of Persons with Disabilities (CRPD), contrasting the medical and social models of disability. This chapter examines the global prevalence of disabilities, focusing on LMICs, where systemic barriers, including inadequate healthcare, poverty, and stigma, exacerbate the challenges faced by individuals with disabilities. Regional analyses highlight disparities in prevalence, with Sub-Saharan Africa, Southeast Asia, and the Middle East bearing disproportionate burdens. This chapter underscores the critical need for inclusive health and education systems to address these inequities, guided by the Sustainable Development Goals (SDGs). By integrating global data and a multidimensional framework, this discussion lays the groundwork for understanding disability as a developmental and human rights issue, advocating for policies that prioritize equity and inclusivity.

1.1 Definitions of Disability (WHO, CRPD)

Disability is a complex and multidimensional concept that can be understood through various frameworks. The World Health Organization (WHO) and the Convention on the Rights of Persons with Disabilities (CRPD) provide widely accepted definitions that help shape the understanding of disability at the global level (Kazou, 2017).

According to the WHO (2021), disability is an umbrella term encompassing impairment, activity limitations, and participation restrictions. This definition is based on the International Classification of Functioning, Disability, and Health (ICF), Fig. 1.1, which recognizes that disability is not just a consequence of an individual's medical condition but also the result of the interaction between health conditions and the environmental and social factors that may impede full participation in society. This model emphasizes the social model of disability, which asserts that disability arises from barriers in society—physical, attitudinal, or environmental—that prevent

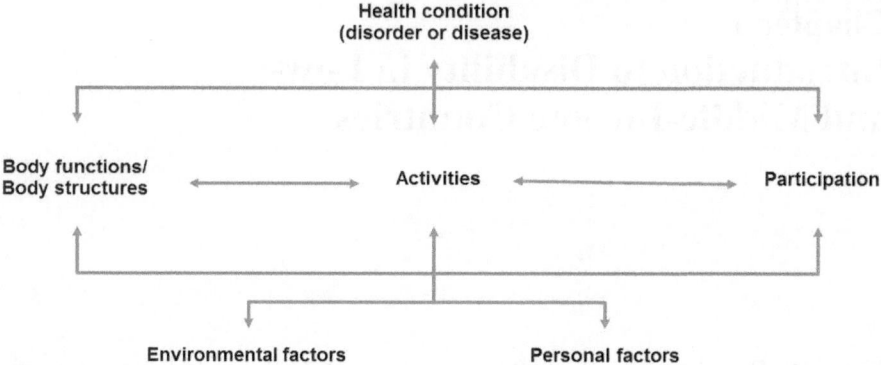

Fig. 1.1 The integrative bio-psycho-social model of functioning, disability, and health (WHO, 2001: 18)

individuals from engaging in normal daily activities rather than being an inherent feature of the individual's body (World Health Organization [WHO], 2021).

- **Impairment** refers to a problem in body function or structure, such as a loss or abnormality in physiological, mental, or anatomical function (WHO, 2021).
- **Activity limitation** refers to difficulties an individual may experience executing tasks or actions (WHO, 2021).
- **Participation restriction** refers to problems an individual may experience when engaging in life situations, such as participating in education, work, or social activities (WHO, 2021).

The social model emphasizes that disability is a consequence of how society is organized. It views disability as a result of societal barriers rather than the individual's impairment. These barriers can include inaccessible environments, discrimination, or lack of accommodation for people with impairments (Shakespeare & Watson, 2001). According to this model, society should be transformed to accommodate individuals with disabilities, promoting inclusion and participation in all aspects of life (Oliver, 1996).

The CRPD (2006), adopted by the United Nations, asserts that disability results from the interaction between individuals with impairments and environmental barriers. It promotes a human rights-based approach, focusing on fully including persons with disabilities in all aspects of society. The CRPD broadens the definition of disability beyond health conditions and includes the impact of social, cultural, and environmental barriers preventing individuals from enjoying the same rights and opportunities. This perspective aligns with the social model of disability, emphasizing removing societal barriers to ensure full participation.

Key definitions from the CRPD include:

- **Persons with Disabilities:** "Those who have long-term physical, mental, intellectual, or sensory impairments which, in interaction with various barriers, may

hinder their full and effective participation in society on an equal basis with others"
(United Nations, 2006).

- **Discrimination based on Disability:** The CRPD explicitly identifies the need
to eliminate discrimination and promote equal participation in societal processes
(United Nations, 2006).

While the medical model views disability as an individual problem that requires
medical treatment or rehabilitation, the social model frames it as a societal issue,
calling for the removal of barriers to ensure full inclusion and participation (Shakespeare & Watson, 2001). The shift from the medical to the social model has been
central to disability rights movements worldwide, leading to policies and frameworks like the CRPD, which advocate for the rights and autonomy of people with
disabilities.

In the context of low- and middle-income countries (LMICs), the emphasis on
the social model of disability is particularly relevant. In these regions, the lack of
infrastructure, healthcare, and social inclusion often exacerbates the marginalization
of people with disabilities. Understanding disability as a social issue—rather than
solely a medical condition—encourages the creation of policies that foster inclusivity
and accessibility (Oliver, 1996).

This chapter, therefore, will define disability from both medical and social
perspectives and highlight the importance of adopting inclusive practices that challenge societal barriers. By embracing the social model, societies can promote equity
and improve the quality of life for individuals with disabilities, especially in LMICs,
where access to resources and opportunities is often limited.

1.2 Global and Regional Prevalence

Disability is a global issue that affects people of all ages, genders, and socioeconomic
backgrounds. The World Health Organization (WHO) estimates that over 1.3 billion
people worldwide, or approximately 16% of the global population, live with some
form of disability (WHO, n.d.). This includes a broad spectrum of physical, sensory,
intellectual, and mental health conditions that can vary in severity, often resulting in
functional limitations and participation restrictions in daily life.

1.2.1 Global Prevalence

The WHO World Report on Disability (2011) highlights that disability is a significant public health and development issue, particularly as populations age globally.
The report emphasizes that disability can affect anyone at any point in their life and
that the prevalence of disability is expected to rise due to aging populations and

the increased prevalence of chronic health conditions, such as diabetes and cardio-vascular diseases (WHO, 2011). The report also notes that certain groups, such as women, older adults, and people living in poverty, are disproportionately affected by disability. Furthermore, disabilities often intersect with other forms of inequality, such as gender, race, and economic status, exacerbating the barriers individuals face in accessing services and opportunities.

1.2.2 Disability in Low- and Middle-Income Countries (LMICs)

While disability is a global issue, its prevalence and impact are particularly pronounced in LMICs. According to the World Bank and UNICEF, people in LMICs are more likely to experience disability due to factors such as inadequate healthcare systems, high rates of infectious diseases, malnutrition, and injuries (UNICEF, 2017; World Bank, 2013). These regions also face significant barriers to disability inclusion, including limited access to rehabilitative services, social stigma, and systemic poverty, which deepen the challenges faced by individuals with disabilities.

1.2.3 Regional Prevalence of Disability in LMICs

The prevalence of disability within LMICs can differ significantly based on regional factors such as healthcare infrastructure, socioeconomic conditions, and public health challenges. For example:

- **Sub-Saharan Africa**: Disability prevalence is particularly high in this region, largely due to high rates of infectious diseases, malnutrition, and limited access to healthcare. The Global Burden of Disease (GBD) study estimates that 10.5% of the population in Sub-Saharan Africa lives with a disability, with higher rates among children and older adults. In this region, disabilities are often compounded by limited access to rehabilitative services and social stigma, creating further barriers to inclusion (Ferrari et al., 2023).
- **Southeast Asia**: In Southeast Asia, the prevalence of disability is estimated to be around 8.7%, with countries like India and Indonesia showing higher rates (Alam et al., 2024). The region's disability burden is heavily influenced by infectious diseases like polio and tuberculosis, as well as traffic accidents, which contribute to a significant number of physical disabilities (Pattnaik et al., 2023). Overall, it is estimated that 1 in every 6 people in Asia and the Pacific—about 690 million people—live with a disability, underlining the significance of addressing disability-related challenges across the region (Crosta & Sanders, 2021).
- **Middle East and North Africa** recorded the highest prevalence (13.1%) (Olusanya et al., 2022).

1.2.4 Comparative Analysis of Disability Prevalence in Children

In examining disability prevalence across various age groups, children and adolescents represent a significant demographic, particularly in LMICs. According to a recent study comparing the prevalence estimates provided by key global health organizations, such as UNICEF and the Global Burden of Disease (GBD) Study, disability in children remains a crucial concern for policymakers. For instance, UNICEF estimates that 28.9 million children aged 0–4 years, and 236.4 million children aged 0–17 years live with moderate-to-severe disabilities, while the GBD study provides slightly different estimates, showing a higher prevalence for children aged under 5 years. These estimates reveal that Sub-Saharan Africa and South Asia are home to a disproportionate number of children with disabilities, underlining the need for comprehensive data to inform policy and intervention programs aimed at improving the lives of children with disabilities globally (Olusanya et al., 2022).

This comparative analysis emphasizes the importance of data alignment across organizations to better understand and address disability prevalence in LMICs. It also underscores the necessity of inclusive health and education systems that can accommodate and support children with disabilities in these regions.

1.2.5 Healthcare Access

In many LMICs, healthcare systems are under-resourced, and people with disabilities often lack access to basic healthcare services, including rehabilitation, mobility aids, and early interventions. The WHO report also highlights the limited availability of specialized healthcare professionals trained to address the needs of individuals with disabilities in many LMICs. This lack of access to healthcare, combined with social and economic exclusion, contributes to the disproportionate burden of disability in these regions (WHO, 2011).

In a systematic review exploring access to general healthcare services for people with disabilities in low and middle-income countries (LMICs), it was found that utilization and healthcare expenditure were higher for individuals with disabilities. The review included studies from sub-Saharan Africa, Latin America, and East Asia/Pacific, highlighting variations in healthcare access. However, the wide variation in disability types and access measures made cross-study comparisons challenging. The authors concluded that developing common metrics for measuring disability and healthcare access could improve the quality of data and monitor healthcare access for people with disabilities more effectively (Bright & Kuper, 2018).

Fig. 1.2 The dimensions of
stigma: societal,
self-directed, and structural

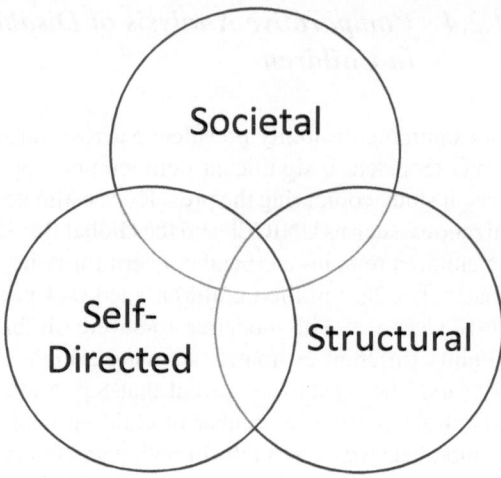

1.2.6 Stigma and Social Exclusion

Stigma and discrimination against people with disabilities are widespread in LMICs, often rooted in cultural beliefs and societal attitudes that view disability as a punishment or a source of shame. As a result, people with disabilities are frequently marginalized in society, facing barriers to education, employment, and social participation. Studies by UNICEF indicate that children with disabilities are particularly vulnerable to exclusion from educational opportunities, leading to a lifetime of disadvantage (UNICEF, 2017).

The global discussion on developmental disabilities (DD) highlights the significant impact of stigma on the lives of affected individuals and their families. Stigma is a complex concept with multiple dimensions, including societal, self-directed, and structural aspects, Fig. 1.2. Societal stigma involves negative perceptions and discriminatory actions from the broader community. In contrast, self-stigma arises when individuals internalize these societal biases, resulting in reduced self-esteem and self-worth. Structural stigma manifests through institutional policies or practices that exclude or disadvantage individuals with disabilities, creating barriers to education, employment, and healthcare access (Link & Phelan, 2001). Sociologist Goffman (1963) explains that stigma occurs when an individual is diminished or viewed negatively because of a perceived characteristic, such as a developmental disability.

1.2.7 Poverty and Disability

The relationship between disability and poverty is bidirectional. On the one hand, people with disabilities are more likely to experience poverty due to barriers to employment, education, and healthcare. On the other hand, living in poverty increases the likelihood of acquiring disabilities, especially in environments where there is limited access to healthcare, sanitation, and safety measures. The World Bank estimates that the economic impact of disability in LMICs is substantial, as it reduces the productivity of individuals and imposes a heavy financial burden on families and communities (World Bank, 2013).

Disability is a global challenge that is particularly pronounced in LMICs, where social, economic, and healthcare barriers exacerbate its impact. Addressing the needs of people with disabilities in these regions requires a comprehensive approach that includes improving healthcare access, reducing stigma, and addressing the structural factors that contribute to inequality. Understanding the global and regional prevalence of disability is essential for developing effective policies and interventions that promote inclusion and equal opportunities for all.

1.3 Types of Disabilities in LMICs

In LMICs, the most prevalent types of disabilities often reflect both medical conditions and socio-environmental factors. The burden of disability is compounded by limited access to essential services such as medical care, rehabilitation, and education, further marginalizing affected individuals. The following are the most common types of disabilities encountered in these regions:

1.3.1 Physical Disabilities

Physical disabilities, including mobility impairments, are among the most common types of disabilities in LMICs. These disabilities can result from congenital conditions, accidents, or diseases such as polio, stroke, or trauma from conflict and natural disasters. Access to appropriate assistive devices like wheelchairs and prosthetics is often limited, exacerbating mobility challenges. In many LMICs, a lack of trained professionals and rehabilitation services leaves individuals with physical disabilities unable to fully integrate into society (WHO, 2011).

1.3.2 Visual and Hearing Impairments

Visual and hearing impairments are prevalent in LMICs due to factors such as lack of early detection, inadequate healthcare infrastructure, and higher rates of preventable conditions like cataracts, glaucoma, and infections. Approximately 80% of the world's visually impaired population lives in LMICs, with a substantial number of these impairments being avoidable through accessible healthcare and early intervention (UNICEF, 2019). Similarly, hearing impairments in LMICs often go undiagnosed or untreated, leading to significant communication barriers and social exclusion, especially in rural areas.

1.3.3 Intellectual Disabilities

Intellectual disabilities (ID), which can include conditions like Down syndrome, autism spectrum disorder (ASD), and other developmental disabilities, are also widespread in LMICs. Studies indicate that the prevalence of ASD is increasing. Still, the lack of specialized educational and therapeutic interventions means that children with intellectual disabilities often do not receive the support they need. This is particularly true in rural and underserved areas where healthcare systems may be underdeveloped (Global Burden of Disease Study, 2017).

1.3.4 Mental Health Disorders

Mental health disabilities, including conditions like depression, anxiety, schizophrenia, and bipolar disorder, are another significant aspect of disability in LMICs. Mental health services are generally scarce in these regions, and the stigma associated with mental illness can prevent individuals from seeking treatment. The social stigma surrounding mental health disorders often leads to isolation, while poverty and lack of access to care exacerbate the severity of these conditions (World Bank, 2020).

1.4 Compounding Factors

Several factors often magnify the burden of these disabilities in LMICs:

- **Lack of Access to Medical Care**: Limited healthcare infrastructure and a shortage of healthcare professionals prevent individuals with disabilities from receiving timely diagnosis, treatment, and rehabilitation services (Bright & Kuper, 2018).
- **Inadequate Rehabilitation Services**: Rehabilitation programs, including physical therapy, speech therapy, and occupational therapy, are frequently underdeveloped or absent in LMICs. As a result, many individuals with disabilities do not achieve the level of functioning they could with proper rehabilitation (Marasinghe et al., 2015).

- **Educational Barriers**: Education systems in LMICs often do not accommodate students with disabilities. The lack of inclusive education policies and the physical inaccessibility of schools further marginalize disabled children, limiting their future opportunities for employment and social participation (UNESCO, 2014).

1.5   The Importance of Addressing Disability in LMICs

Addressing disability in LMICs is not only a matter of humanitarian concern but is also integral to broader economic and social development. People with disabilities often face exclusion from various aspects of life, including education, employment, and social participation, which perpetuates cycles of poverty and inequality. Failing to integrate individuals with disabilities into societal frameworks undermines efforts to foster inclusive growth and development.

Sustainable Development Goals (SDGs) provide a crucial framework for addressing disability-related challenges. Specifically, Goal 10: Reduced Inequality and Goal 4: Quality Education underscore the necessity of inclusion in all areas of society. Goal 10 calls for reducing inequality within and among countries, including targeting the systemic marginalization faced by people with disabilities. Goal 4 highlights the importance of ensuring inclusive education, noting that quality education for all, including individuals with disabilities, is essential for sustainable development (United Nations, 2015).

People with disabilities in LMICs often encounter substantial barriers that limit their access to education and employment. This exclusion exacerbates poverty by hindering individuals' ability to earn income, while the lack of access to quality education perpetuates disparities in opportunities. The World Bank has highlighted that disability is both a cause and a consequence of poverty, as individuals with disabilities often face significant challenges accessing employment, healthcare, and social services, leading to a higher likelihood of living in poverty (World Bank, 2018).

Moreover, exclusion from the labor market and education further entrenches the economic vulnerability of individuals with disabilities, limiting their potential to contribute to the economy and benefit from its growth. The United Nations Convention on the Rights of Persons with Disabilities (CRPD) emphasizes that persons with disabilities must enjoy the same opportunities as others in education, employment, and social participation (United Nations, 2006). This framework advocates for a shift toward inclusive practices that recognize the capacities of people with disabilities and remove the societal barriers that hinder their participation ilities, is essential for sustainable development.(United Nations, 2015).

Implementing policies that guarantee access to quality education and employment for people with disabilities and ensure their full participation in social, economic, and political life is essential to promoting inclusive development.

1.6   Conclusion

The prevalence of disabilities in LMICs is substantial, and the types of disabilities most commonly found include physical disabilities, visual and hearing impairments, intellectual disabilities, and mental health disorders. Addressing these issues requires comprehensive efforts to improve access to healthcare, rehabilitation, and education. These efforts should focus on overcoming societal and environmental barriers that prevent individuals with disabilities from fully participating in society.

References

Alam, M. B., Khanam, S. J., Rana, M. S., Khandaker, G., Kabir, M. A., & Khan, M. N. (2024). Effects of disability on adverse health outcomes and anthropometric deficits among under-five children in South Asian countries: Evidence from multiple indicator cluster surveys. *The Lancet Regional Health-Southeast Asia, 25*, 100401. https://doi.org/10.1016/j.lansea.2024.100401

Bright, T., & Kuper, H. (2018). A systematic review of access to general healthcare services for people with disabilities in low and middle income countries. *International Journal of Environmental Research and Public Health, 15*(9), 1879. https://doi.org/10.3390/ijerph150 91879

Crosta, N., & Sanders, A. (2021). Overview: Disability in the ASEAN region. In N. Crosta & A. Sanders (Eds.), *Social enterprises and disability: Fostering innovation, awareness, and social impact in the ASEAN region* (pp. 1–7). ERIA.

Ferrari, A. J., et al. (2023). Global incidence, prevalence, years lived with disability (YLDs), disability-adjusted life-years (DALYs), and healthy life expectancy (HALE) for 371 diseases and injuries in 204 countries and territories and 811 subnational locations, 1990–2021: A systematic analysis for the Global Burden of Disease Study 2021. *The Lancet, 403*(10440), 2133–2161.

Global Burden of Disease Study (GBD). (2017). *Disability-Adjusted Life Years (DALYs) and years lived with disability (YLDs) estimates.* http://www.healthdata.org/gbd/2017

Goffman, E. (1963). *Stigma: Notes on the management of spoiled identity.* Prentice-Hall. https://bac-lac.on.worldcat.org/oclc/223060

Kazou, K. (2017). Analysing the definition of disability in the UN convention on the rights of persons with disabilities: Is it really based on a 'social model' approach? *International Journal of Mental Health and Capacity Law, 23*, 25–48. https://doi.org/10.19164/ijmhcl.v2017i23.630.

Link, B. G., & Phelan, J. C. (2001). Conceptualizing stigma. *Annual Review of Sociology, 27*, 363–385.

Marasinghe, K. M., Lapitan, J. M., & Ross, A. (2015). Assistive technologies for ageing populations in six low-income and middle-income countries: A systematic review. *BMJ Innovations, 1*(4), 182–195. https://doi.org/10.1136/bmjinnov-2015-000065

Oliver, M. (1996). Understanding disability: From theory to practice. *The Journal of Sociology & Social Welfare, 23*(3), Article 24. https://doi.org/10.15453/0191-5096.2372. https://scholarwo rks.wmich.edu/jssw/vol23/iss3/24

Olusanya, B. O., Kancherla, V., Shaheen, A., Ogbo, F. A., & Davis, A. C. (2022). Global and regional prevalence of disabilities among children and adolescents: Analysis of findings from global health databases. *Frontiers in Public Health, 10*, 977453. https://doi.org/10.3389/fpubh. 2022.977453

Pattnaik, S., Murmu, J., Agrawal, R., Rehman, T., Kanungo, S., & Pati, S. (2023). Prevalence, pattern and determinants of disabilities in India: Insights from NFHS-5 (2019–21). *Frontiers in Public Health, 11*, 1036499. https://doi.org/10.3389/fpubh.2023.1036499

Shakespeare, T., & Watson, N. (2001). The social model of disability: An outdated ideology? In S. N. Barnartt & B. M. Altman (Ed.), *Exploring theories and expanding methodologies: Where we are and where we need to go* (Research in Social Science and Disability, Vol. 2, pp. 9–28). Emerald Group Publishing Limited. https://doi.org/10.1016/S1479-3547(01)80018-X

UNESCO. (2014). *Teaching and learning: Achieving quality for all* (EFA Global Monitoring Report 2014). UNESCO. http://www.uis.unesco.org/Library/Documents/gmr-2013-14-teaching-and-learning-education-for-all-2014-en.pdf

UNICEF. (2017). *Disability in the context of children and adolescents: A rights-based perspective.* https://www.unicef.org/reports/disability-rights-children

UNICEF. (2019). *The state of the world's children 2019: Children with disabilities.* https://www.unicef.org/reports/state-of-worlds-children-2019

United Nations. (2006). *Convention on the Rights of Persons with Disabilities (CRPD).* https://www.un.org/disabilities/documents/convention/convoptprotections.pdf

United Nations. (2015). *Sustainable development goals (SDGs).* https://sdgs.un.org/goals

World Bank. (2013). *Disability and development: A World Bank group strategy.* World Bank Group. https://openknowledge.worldbank.org/handle/10986/16817

World Bank. (2018). *Disability inclusion in development: The case for change.* https://www.worldbank.org/en/topic/disability

World Bank. (2020). *World development report 2020: Disability inclusion.* https://www.worldbank.org/en/publication/wdr2020

World Health Organization. (n.d.). *Disability and health.* World Health Organization. https://www.who.int/news-room/fact-sheets/detail/disability-and-health

World Health Organization. (2001). *The International Classification of Functioning, Disability and Health (ICF).* Geneva: WHO. http://www.who.int/classifications/icf/en/

World Health Organization. (WHO). (2011). *World report on disability.* WHO Press. https://www.who.int/disabilities/world_report/2011/en/

World Health Organization. (WHO). (2021). *World report on disability.* World Health Organization. https://www.who.int/publications/i/item/world-report-on-disability

Chapter 2
Healthcare Access for People with Disabilities in LMICs

Abstract In low- and middle-income countries (LMICs), people with disabilities encounter complex barriers to healthcare access, including economic constraints, physical inaccessibility, and societal stigma. These challenges exacerbate health inequities and limit opportunities for achieving optimal well-being. This chapter explores the prevalence and multifaceted impact of disability in LMICs, highlighting the cyclical relationship between poverty, exclusion, and poor health outcomes. Drawing on theoretical frameworks such as the Social Model of Disability and the Capability Approach, this chapter examines systemic barriers and their far-reaching implications. It emphasizes the importance of international policies, including the United Nations Convention on the Rights of Persons with Disabilities (CRPD) and the Sustainable Development Goals (SDGs), in fostering disability-inclusive healthcare systems. Promising strategies such as community-based rehabilitation programs, infrastructure improvements, and the integration of assistive technologies demonstrate the potential for transformative change. However, significant gaps persist in knowledge and implementation, underscoring the need for robust, context-specific research. This chapter invites a call to action for stakeholders to develop innovative, sustainable approaches that advance equity and inclusivity in healthcare for individuals with disabilities in LMICs.

2.1 The Prevalence and Impact of Disability in LMICs

Globally, an estimated one billion people, or 15% of the population, live with some form of disability, with the highest prevalence found in LMICs. The United Nations Convention on the Rights of Persons with Disabilities (CRPD) highlights the need for full societal inclusion and access to healthcare for individuals with disabilities. However, individuals with disabilities in LMICs face compound challenges. Poverty, malnutrition, and lack of access to basic services often lead to increased vulnerability to disability, which, in turn, exacerbates economic disadvantage (World Bank, 2023). Studies show that people with disabilities in these regions are more likely to experience adverse socioeconomic outcomes, such as lower educational attainment, poor

A. Al Shami and A. J. Nashwan, *Global Health and Disability*,
SpringerBriefs in Modern Perspectives on Disability Research,
https://doi.org/10.1007/978-981-96-4956-3_2

health outcomes, and higher poverty rates, further limiting their access to essential healthcare (World Bank, 2023).

In LMICs, disability is not only a health issue but a multifaceted social issue. Access to education, employment, and healthcare is often limited due to systemic barriers, including physical inaccessibility, inadequate assistive devices, and discriminatory societal attitudes. Consequently, people with disabilities experience greater social isolation and poorer health outcomes, which in turn contribute to a cycle of poverty and limited access to healthcare services (Nussbaum, 2011).

2.2   Key Barriers to Healthcare Access

Economic, physical, and social barriers significantly hinder healthcare access for people with disabilities in low- and middle-income countries (LMICs). These challenges encompass financial constraints, inadequate infrastructure, and societal stigma, all of which exacerbate healthcare inequities, Fig. 2.1.

2.2.1   Economic Barriers

Economic barriers are among the most significant obstacles to healthcare access for people with disabilities in LMICs. Many individuals with disabilities live in poverty, making healthcare unaffordable. Direct costs such as medical fees, mobility aids, assistive devices, and medications are often prohibitive (Marasinghe et al., 2015). Moreover, indirect costs, such as lost income due to disability or caregiving responsibilities, further strain families already living in poverty. These economic challenges often prevent individuals from seeking timely medical intervention, exacerbating health conditions (Clemente et al., 2022).

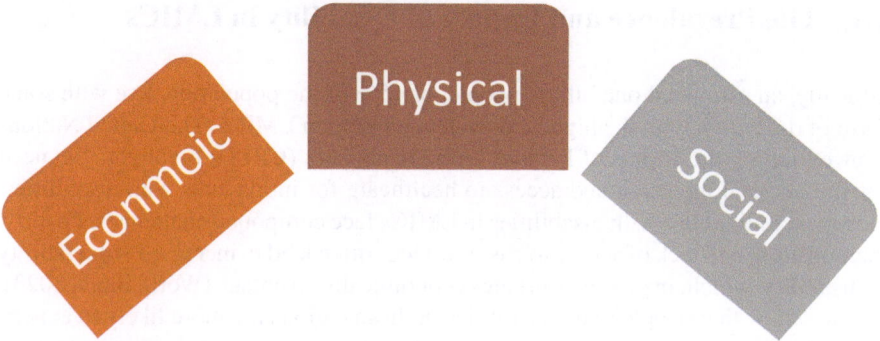

Fig. 2.1 Key barriers to healthcare access for people with disabilities in LMICs

Addressing these economic challenges is crucial for improving healthcare access in LMICs. Developing common metrics for measuring disability and healthcare access, as well as implementing interventions aimed at increasing access to health services for vulnerable populations, are essential steps toward achieving equitable healthcare access (Bright et al., 2017).

2.2.2 Physical and Infrastructure Barriers

The lack of accessible healthcare infrastructure is another critical barrier. Many healthcare facilities in LMICs are not designed to accommodate individuals with disabilities. This includes a lack of ramps, accessible toilets, and specialized equipment, making it difficult or even impossible for people with mobility impairments to access healthcare (Cote, 2021). Furthermore, transportation remains a significant challenge in rural areas, where public transport systems are often inadequate or inaccessible, further limiting access to healthcare services (WHO, 2011).

A qualitative study conducted in the Luuka district of Uganda further highlights these challenges, revealing interconnected barriers that impede equitable healthcare access for persons with disabilities. The study reported that inaccessible healthcare facilities, often lacking features like ramps and other accessibility modifications, compounded the difficulties faced by individuals with mobility and sensory impairments. Moreover, the absence of healthcare workers and frequent service delivery delays were common, exacerbating the issue of poor care. The findings emphasize the urgent need for systemic changes to healthcare infrastructure and service delivery to ensure that healthcare facilities meet the diverse needs of all individuals, including those with disabilities (Ssemata et al., 2024).

2.2.3 Social and Cultural Barriers

Social stigma and cultural attitudes toward people with disabilities also impede healthcare access. Negative perceptions often lead to discrimination, marginalization, and exclusion of individuals with disabilities from healthcare services. Health providers in LMICs may lack the training and awareness needed to effectively address the needs of people with disabilities, further perpetuating this exclusion (Hashemi et al., 2022). Furthermore, the lack of accessible information about health conditions, prevention strategies, and treatments, especially for those with sensory disabilities (e.g., visual or hearing impairments), exacerbates the challenges faced by this population (Eleweke & Ebenso, 2016).

Gender disparities add another layer to these social and cultural barriers. A study on women and girls with disabilities in Lebanon revealed significant challenges in accessing healthcare services, with females constituting only 33.4% of users in a

humanitarian physical rehabilitation program. Beyond common barriers like inadequate infrastructure and financial constraints, women faced unique challenges rooted
in societal norms. These included safety concerns during unaccompanied visits to
healthcare facilities, economic disparities, and preferences for female healthcare
providers to ensure privacy. The findings underscore the importance of addressing
gender-specific barriers and implementing targeted interventions to promote equity
in healthcare access (Abou-Abbas et al., 2024).

2.3   Frameworks for Understanding Healthcare Access Barriers

This section explores key frameworks for understanding healthcare access barriers
faced by individuals with disabilities, focusing on the Social Model of Disability
and the Capability Approach. Both frameworks provide essential insights into
addressing systemic barriers and promoting inclusive healthcare for people with
disabilities.

2.3.1   The Social Model of Disability

The social model of disability provides a critical lens for understanding the barriers
to healthcare faced by individuals with disabilities. This model posits that disability
is not solely the result of an individual's impairments but is primarily caused by
societal barriers that limit participation in various aspects of life, including healthcare (Mahmoud et al., 2022). According to this framework, society is responsible
for removing these barriers and creating an environment where all individuals can
access healthcare services. The social model highlights the importance of addressing
systemic issues such as physical inaccessibility, societal stigma, and the lack of
inclusive healthcare infrastructure (Baart & Taaka, 2017).

2.3.2   The Capability Approach

As outlined by Nussbaum (2011), the capability approach offers a valuable perspective on healthcare access for people with disabilities. This framework emphasizes
the need to expand the capabilities of individuals, allowing them to lead lives they
have reason to value, which includes the ability to access quality healthcare. In
the context of LMICs, the capability approach advocates for ensuring that people
with disabilities can achieve the necessary functioning in health, education, and

employment by removing barriers that prevent their full participation in society (Vergunst et al., 2017).

2.4   The Role of International Policy in Improving Healthcare Access

International policies, such as the United Nations Convention on the Rights of Persons with Disabilities (CRPD), play a crucial role in promoting the rights of people with disabilities and improving healthcare access in LMICs. The CRPD, ratified by 185 countries, specifically calls for integrating people with disabilities into all aspects of society, including healthcare (World Bank, 2023). This includes ensuring access to healthcare services and assistive devices and removing barriers to healthcare delivery.

The 2030 Agenda for Sustainable Development, which includes the Sustainable Development Goals (SDGs), further emphasizes the need for disability-inclusive development. The SDGs incorporate targets that directly address the needs of people with disabilities, particularly health and well-being. These international frameworks provide a roadmap for improving healthcare access and achieving greater equity for individuals with disabilities (Adugna et al., 2020).

Additionally, international policy can play a critical role in addressing the growing unmet need for rehabilitation services in LMICs. Despite urgent calls for action, many governments in these regions have given little attention to expanding rehabilitation services. A policy framework developed through key informant interviews across 47 countries highlighted three key barriers to prioritizing rehabilitation on national health agendas: a lack of consistent problem definition, fragmented governance arrangements, and national legacies such as those stemming from civil conflict. These barriers undermine the development of effective solutions for advancing rehabilitation services and improving healthcare access for people with disabilities. Addressing these barriers at the policy level is essential to improve equity in access to rehabilitation and ensure that rehabilitation is appropriately prioritized in LMICs (Neill et al., 2023).

2.5   Strategies for Enhancing Healthcare Access for People with Disabilities in Low- and Middle-Income Countries

This section discusses key strategies for improving healthcare access for people with disabilities in low- and middle-income countries (LMICs). It highlights the importance of policy development, infrastructure improvements, and training healthcare providers to meet the diverse needs of individuals with disabilities.

2.5.1 Policy Development and Advocacy

Effective policy development is essential to improving healthcare access for people with disabilities, particularly in low- and middle-income countries (LMICs). Policy-makers in LMICs must prioritize disability inclusion in national healthcare strategies and ensure that healthcare systems are equipped to meet the needs of individuals with disabilities. Advocacy efforts at the local, national, and international levels are critical in pushing for changes to existing policies and promoting the implementation of the Convention on the Rights of Persons with Disabilities (CRPD) and Sustainable Development Goals (SDGs) (Matter et al., 2017). For example, the WHO Global Disability Action Plan (2014–2021) encourages LMICs to integrate disability into health systems and policies, promoting equitable healthcare access for all (World Health Organization, 2014). In countries like India, the National Disability Insurance Scheme (NDIS) offers tailored support for people with disabilities, ensuring they have access to healthcare services (National Disability Insurance Agency, 2020). Furthermore, countries such as Uganda and Kenya have used the CRPD to guide national health policy reforms that focus on improving healthcare access for people with disabilities, addressing issues such as physical accessibility, health literacy, and healthcare coverage (United Nations, 2006).

2.5.2 Improving Healthcare Infrastructure

Improving the physical infrastructure of healthcare facilities is essential to ensuring accessibility for people with disabilities in LMICs. Many healthcare facilities in LMICs lack basic accessibility features, which further restricts access for individuals with mobility impairments, sensory impairments, and other disabilities. Retrofitting existing healthcare facilities to meet accessibility standards and constructing new ones with universal design principles can significantly improve healthcare access. For example, the World Bank has supported initiatives in countries like Ethiopia and Tanzania to improve healthcare infrastructure, ensuring that medical facilities are designed to be accessible to people with disabilities (World Bank, 2022). In addition, the provision of necessary assistive devices, such as wheelchairs and hearing aids, is crucial. Community-based healthcare programs in LMICs have proven to be effective in bridging the healthcare gap, especially in rural and remote areas. For example, community health worker programs in India have been successful in providing primary healthcare services, disability identification, and referrals to specialized care (Bhatia, 2014). These programs allow healthcare access to populations that would otherwise be underserved due to geographical or financial barriers.

2.5.3 Education and Training for Healthcare Providers

Training healthcare professionals in LMICs to understand the diverse needs of people with disabilities is crucial to improving healthcare outcomes. Many healthcare providers in LMICs lack formal training on disability, which can result in misdiagnoses, inadequate care, and the perpetuation of stigma. Healthcare training programs in LMICs should focus on addressing the physical, communication, and psychological needs of patients with disabilities, ensuring that they receive equitable and effective care. In countries like Zambia, the World Health Organization (WHO) has collaborated with local governments to provide disability-inclusive health training for healthcare workers, enhancing their ability to serve people with disabilities (World Health Organization, 2021). The integration of disability awareness in the medical curricula of universities in South Africa and Uganda has also improved healthcare provider competence in caring for individuals with various disabilities (NHS, 2022). Furthermore, international initiatives, such as the CDC's Disability Health Program in the U.S., have shared best practices in disability-inclusive healthcare, which are being adopted in LMICs to ensure comprehensive care for patients with disabilities (CDC, 2020).

2.6 Conclusion

In conclusion, people with disabilities in LMICs face multiple barriers to accessing healthcare, including economic, physical, social, and attitudinal challenges. These barriers prevent individuals from receiving the necessary care, resulting in poorer health outcomes and greater marginalization. However, frameworks such as the social model of disability and the capability approach provide valuable insights into how these barriers can be addressed. By prioritizing policy development, improving healthcare infrastructure, and training healthcare providers, LMICs can make significant strides in improving healthcare access for people with disabilities. As global awareness of disability-inclusive development grows, there is hope that the healthcare needs of people with disabilities will be met more equitably and comprehensively.

References

Abou-Abbas, L., Sabbagh, D., Rossi, R., Vijayasingham, L., Lteif, M. R., Rawi, H., Mitri, R., Al Sultan, H., Benyaich, A., Al-Mosa, A., & Truppa, C. (2024). Challenges in accessing health care services for women and girls with disabilities using a humanitarian physical rehabilitation program in Lebanon: A mixed method study. *International Journal for Equity in Health, 23*, 267. https://doi.org/10.1186/s12939-024-02356-4
Adugna, M. B., Nabbouh, F., Shehata, S., & Ghahari, S. (2020). Barriers to healthcare access for people with disabilities in low- and middle-income countries: A systematic review. *BMC Health Services Research, 20*, 15. https://doi.org/10.1186/s12913-019-4822-6

Baart, J., & Taaka, F. (2017). Barriers to healthcare services for people with disabilities in developing countries: A literature review. *Asia Pacific Disability Rehabilitation Journal, 29*(4), 26–40. https://doi.org/10.5463/DCID.v29i4.656

Bhatia, K. (2014). Community health worker programs in India: A rights-based review. *Perspectives in Public Health, 134*(5), 276–282. https://doi.org/10.1177/1757913914543446

Bright, T., Felix, L., Kuper, H., & Polack, S. (2017). A systematic review of strategies to increase access to health services among children in low and middle income countries. *BMC Health Services Research, 17*, 252. https://doi.org/10.1186/s12913-017-2180-9

Centers for Disease Control and Prevention (CDC). (2020). *Disability health program.* https://www.cdc.gov/disability-and-health/?CDC_AAref_Val=https://www.cdc.gov/ncbddd/disabilityandhealth/in

Clemente, K. A. P., Silva, S. V., Vieira, G. I., Bortoli, M. C., Toma, T. S., Ramos, V. D., & Brito, C. M. M. D. (2022). Barriers to the access of people with disabilities to health services: A scoping review. *Revista de saude publica, 56*, 64. https://doi.org/10.11606/s1518-8787.2022056003893

Cote, A. (2021). Social protection and access to assistive technology in low- and middle-income countries. *Assistive Technology, 33*(sup1), S102–S108. https://doi.org/10.1080/10400435.2021.1994052

Eleweke, C. J., & Ebenso, J. (2016). Barriers to accessing services by people with disabilities in Nigeria: Insights from a qualitative study. *Journal of Educational and Social Research, 6*(2), 113.

Hashemi, G., Wickenden, M., Bright, T., & Kuper, H. (2022). Barriers to accessing primary healthcare services for people with disabilities in low and middle-income countries: A meta-synthesis of qualitative studies. *Disability and Rehabilitation, 44*(8), 1207–1220. https://doi.org/10.1080/09638288.2020.1817984

Mahmoud, K., Jaramillo, C., & Barteit, S. (2022). Telemedicine in low- and middle-income countries during the COVID-19 pandemic: A scoping review. *Frontiers in Public Health, 10*, 914423. https://doi.org/10.3389/fpubh.2022.914423

Marasinghe, K. M., Lapitan, J. M., & Ross, A. (2015). Assistive technologies for aging populations in six low-income and middle-income countries: A systematic review. *BMJ Innovations, 1*(4), 182–195. https://doi.org/10.1136/bmjinnov-2015-000065

Matter, R., Harniss, M., Oderud, T., Borg, J., & Eide, A. H. (2017). Assistive technology in resource-limited environments: A scoping review. *Disability and Rehabilitation: Assistive Technology, 12*(2), 105–114. https://doi.org/10.1080/17483107.2016.1188170

National Disability Insurance Agency. (2020). *National Disability Insurance Scheme (NDIS).* https://www.ndis.gov.au

National Health Service (NHS). (2022). *Disability awareness in medical training.* https://www.nhs.uk

Neill, R., Shawar, Y. R., Ashraf, L., Das, P., Champagne, S. N., Kautsar, H., Zia, N., Michlig, G. N., & Bachani, A. M. (2023). Prioritizing rehabilitation in low- and middle-income country national health systems: A qualitative thematic synthesis and development of a policy framework. *International Journal for Equity in Health, 22*, 91. https://doi.org/10.1186/s12939-023-01896-5

Nussbaum, M. (2011). *Creating capabilities: The human development approach.* Harvard University Press.

Ssemata, A. S., Smythe, T., Sande, S., Menya, A., Hameed, S., Waiswa, P., & Kuper, H. (2024). Exploring the barriers to healthcare access among persons with disabilities: A qualitative study in rural Luuka district, Uganda. *BMJ Open, 14*, e086194. https://doi.org/10.1136/bmjopen-2024-086194

United Nations. (2006). *Convention on the rights of persons with disabilities.* https://www.un.org/disabilities/documents/convention/convoptprot-e.pdf

Vergunst, R., Swartz, L., Hem, K. G., Eide, A. H., Mannan, H., MacLachlan, M., Mji, G., Braathen, S. H., & Schneider, M. (2017). Barriers to healthcare access for people with disabilities: A systematic review. *BMC Health Services Research, 17*, 741. https://doi.org/10.1186/s12913-017-2674-5

World Bank. (2022, December 14). *Vulnerable Ethiopians to benefit from $745 million in grants for improved access to health services and flood management.* World Bank. https://www.worldbank.org/en/news/press-release/2022/12/14/vulnerable-ethiopians-to-benefit-from-745-million-in-grants-for-improved-access-to-health-services-and-flood-management

World Bank. (2023). *Disability overview.* https://worldbank.org/en/topic/disability

World Health Organization. (2011). *World report on disability.* World Health Organization. https://www.who.int/disabilities/world_report/2011/report.pdf

World Health Organization. (2014). *WHO global disability action plan 2014–2021: Better health for all people with disability.* World Health Organization. https://iris.who.int/bitstream/handle/10665/199544/9789241509619_eng.pdf?sequence=1

World Health Organization. (2021). *Disability-inclusive health training.* https://www.who.int/disabilities

Chapter 3
Educational Inclusion for People with Disabilities in LMICs

Abstract Educational inclusion for individuals with disabilities in low- and middle-income countries (LMICs) remains a critical challenge despite global efforts to ensure access to quality education for all. This chapter explores the barriers impeding educational inclusion in LMICs, including physical, social, economic, and policy-related factors. It examines the effectiveness of inclusive education policies, the outcomes of various educational interventions, and the gaps in existing research. While international frameworks like the UN Sustainable Development Goal (SDG 4) and the Convention on the Rights of Persons with Disabilities (CRPD) advocate for inclusive education, the implementation in LMICs faces significant hurdles such as insufficient resources, societal stigma, and inadequate infrastructure. Policies promoting inclusive education are often underfunded and poorly implemented, exacerbating disparities, especially between urban and rural areas. Despite these challenges, educational interventions in some regions have shown improvements in academic performance, social integration, and employment outcomes for students with disabilities. However, the lack of standardized evaluation methods and long-term studies limits a comprehensive understanding of these interventions' impact. This chapter calls for increased investment in education systems, better resource allocation, and robust research to improve educational outcomes for students with disabilities in LMICs.

3.1 Context of Educational Inclusion in LMICs

- **Global Frameworks**:
  International commitments such as the United Nations Sustainable Development Goal (SDG 4) and the Convention on the Rights of Persons with Disabilities (CRPD) emphasize providing inclusive and equitable education for all. These frameworks advocate for removing barriers to education, ensuring access to learning for people with disabilities, and promoting equality in education systems worldwide (United Nations Development Programme, 2024). They have shaped policy and influence grassroots movements, focusing on ensuring that education is both accessible and inclusive. In LMICs, these frameworks have sparked national

A. Al Shami and A. J. Nashwan, *Global Health and Disability*,
SpringerBriefs in Modern Perspectives on Disability Research,
https://doi.org/10.1007/978-981-96-4956-3_3

reforms, encouraging countries to integrate inclusive practices into their education systems. For example, countries like Kenya and India have initiated policies to promote inclusive education, but challenges such as inadequate resources, cultural stigma, and lack of trained educators still hinder full implementation. These global frameworks continue to drive efforts to remove these barriers, ensuring that students with disabilities can access schools and experience high-quality education that meets their diverse needs.

- **Regional Overview**:

    Socioeconomic factors, including poverty and limited resource access, influence educational inclusion in LMICs. Cultural and political barriers also play a significant role, as education systems in these regions are often underfunded and fragmented, with societal attitudes toward disability varying widely. Common challenges include a lack of trained teachers, inaccessible school infrastructure, and inadequate assistive technologies (Eleweke, 1999; Mariga et al., 2014). For example, in regions like Sub-Saharan Africa, the cultural stigma surrounding disabilities often leads to the social exclusion of students from schools despite policies supporting inclusive education (World Bank, 2020). Furthermore, UNESCO highlights that 40% of low and lower-middle-income countries did not provide specific support to disadvantaged learners during school closures, exacerbating educational disparities. Underfunding of education systems results in large class sizes, limited teaching materials, and insufficient support services, hindering the inclusion of children with disabilities (UNESCO, 2021). Additionally, physical barriers such as inaccessible infrastructure further limit access to education for students with disabilities, as noted by the World Bank (2020). The shortage of trained teachers to address diverse learning needs remains a significant obstacle, with studies emphasizing the need for systemic reforms and capacity-building initiatives to enhance inclusive education (RTI International, 2022; UNESCO, 2021). Limited access to assistive technologies also hampers the educational experiences of children with disabilities in LMICs. Addressing these challenges requires comprehensive policies, adequate funding, and a cultural shift to reduce stigma and promote inclusivity.

3.2 Barriers to Education for People with Disabilities in LMICs

The barriers to education for children with disabilities in Low- and Middle-Income Countries (LMICs) are multifaceted, encompassing physical, social, economic, and policy-related challenges. These obstacles not only prevent children with disabilities from accessing education, but also perpetuate exclusion and inequality, limiting their opportunities for personal development and future success. The following sections delve into these key barriers, providing a comprehensive overview of how they impact the educational participation of students with disabilities in LMICs. Table 3.1 summarizes the different categories of barriers and their corresponding effects on students' educational experiences.

- **Physical Barriers**: Many schools in LMICs lack accessible infrastructure, such as ramps, accessible toilets, and assistive technologies, which are crucial for the full participation of students with disabilities. Furthermore, educational materials are often not adapted to meet the diverse needs of learners with disabilities, putting them at a disadvantage (World Health Organization [WHO] & World Bank, 2011). In many rural LMICs, children with mobility impairments are often unable to access school buildings that lack ramps or are located on upper floors, creating significant barriers to education. For example, a report by UNESCO (2019) highlights that less than 10% of schools in some Sub-Saharan African countries meet minimum accessibility standards. Additionally, inadequate transportation infrastructure and long travel distances to schools disproportionately affect children with physical disabilities in rural areas (UNICEF, 2020). The lack of adapted teaching aids, such as braille textbooks or audio-visual materials for students with visual and hearing impairments, further exacerbates the exclusion of students with disabilities from educational opportunities (International Disability Alliance, 2021).
- **Social Barriers**: Social stigma and discrimination are prevalent in many LMICs, where disabilities are often perceived as a source of shame or a sign of inferiority. This stigma leads to the exclusion of children with disabilities from mainstream education and reinforces negative stereotypes. Additionally, teachers often lack the training and resources to effectively teach children with disabilities (Sightsavers, 2021). Beyond discrimination within schools, societal stigma frequently deters families from enrolling their children with disabilities, as they fear the

Table 3.1 Summary of barriers to education for children with disabilities in LMICs

Barrier type	Description	Key Examples
Physical Barriers	Lack of accessible infrastructure and teaching aids for students with disabilities	Lack of ramps, inaccessible school buildings, absence of adapted materials (e.g., Braille, audio-visual aids)
Social Barriers	Stigma and discrimination in both schools and communities that prevent full integration of students with disabilities	Societal stigma, bullying, negative stereotypes, reluctance of families to enroll children with disabilities
Economic Barriers	High costs of education and support services, making access difficult for families in poverty	School fees, transportation costs, lack of assistive devices and specialized teachers
Policy/Systemic Barriers	Weak implementation of inclusive education policies due to insufficient resources and political will	Inconsistent policy application, lack of monitoring, inadequate funding for necessary resources

social repercussions and isolation that may follow. A study by the World Bank (2018) highlights that in many communities, children with disabilities are seen as a financial burden or as unworthy of education, further contributing to their exclusion from educational opportunities. Moreover, research by the Global Partnership for Education (2020) found that negative societal attitudes often lead to higher dropout rates among children with disabilities, as parents are reluctant to send their children to schools where they may face bullying or social ostracism.

- **Economic Barriers**: In LMICs, the cost of education—such as school fees, transportation, and the provision of specialized support services—can be prohibitive for families living in poverty. Economic hardships prevent many families from sending their children with disabilities to school, limiting access to education and future opportunities (WHO & World Bank, 2011). For example, a report by the Global Partnership for Education (2020) highlights that families in rural areas often struggle with the costs of transportation to schools that may be located far from their homes, further exacerbating barriers to education for children with disabilities. Additionally, the lack of financial resources makes it difficult for schools to provide necessary support services, such as specialized teachers or assistive devices, which are essential for the inclusion of children with disabilities in mainstream education (UNICEF, 2019). As a result, children with disabilities are frequently left behind in terms of education, perpetuating cycles of poverty and marginalization.
- **Policy and Systemic Barriers**: Despite inclusive education policies in many LMICs, weak implementation and a lack of government funding often undermine their effectiveness. Insufficient monitoring mechanisms, combined with limited accountability and political will, hinder the creation of inclusive education systems (Hayes & Bulat, 2017; Mariga et al., 2014). For instance, the Global Partnership for Education (2018) reports that, even in countries with established policies for inclusive education, many schools continue to lack the resources and infrastructure needed to implement these policies effectively. Additionally, a study by the World Bank (2020) emphasized that insufficient training for policymakers and educators, alongside poor coordination between national and local education authorities, has led to inconsistent policy implementation across different regions. Furthermore, the lack of financial and human resources dedicated to disability inclusion in education exacerbates these barriers, preventing meaningful change (UNESCO, 2021).

These barriers collectively contribute to the marginalization of children with disabilities, limiting their opportunities for education and perpetuating cycles of inequality. Table 3.1 provides an overview of these barriers and their impact on students' access to education.

3.3 Effectiveness of Inclusive Education Policies

Inclusive education policies in LMICs have made significant strides, aligning more closely with international frameworks such as the CRPD and SDG 4. However, the success of these policies is heavily dependent on political commitment, adequate resource allocation, and overcoming challenges in implementation to ensure effective education for children with disabilities.

- **Policy Landscape**: National policies in LMICs, while varied, are increasingly aligned with international frameworks such as the CRPD and SDG 4. These frameworks emphasize the right of children with disabilities to receive an inclusive education, ensuring that they are not segregated from their peers and have equal opportunities to participate in mainstream education. Countries like Kenya and India have made significant strides in establishing inclusive education policies, but challenges remain regarding nationwide coverage and quality. For example, despite Kenya's national policy on inclusive education, there are disparities in access between urban and rural areas, with urban schools generally better equipped to meet the needs of students with disabilities (United Nations, 2017). Political commitment, coupled with proper resource allocation, is essential for the successful implementation of these policies.
- **Implementation Challenges**: The effectiveness of inclusive education policies in LMICs often suffers from challenges in resource allocation. These challenges include a lack of trained teachers, insufficient funding for infrastructure improvements, and inadequate provision of necessary assistive devices and technologies. Furthermore, integrating children with disabilities into regular classrooms without appropriate support mechanisms often leads to poor educational outcomes. Teachers may lack the necessary skills to manage diverse classrooms effectively, and schools may not be adequately equipped to accommodate the physical and educational needs of students with disabilities. In countries like India, while inclusive education policies exist, gaps in resources and teacher training undermine their effectiveness (Mariga et al., 2014). International aid and partnerships with NGOs are crucial in bridging these gaps. NGOs provide support for infrastructure improvements, teacher training, and the distribution of assistive devices, which are critical for ensuring that children with disabilities have the necessary resources to succeed in education. However, long-term sustainability remains a significant challenge, as reliance on external support may not provide a permanent solution. Effective policy implementation requires not only international collaboration but also sustained national investment in education systems.

The continuous evaluation of inclusive education policies and programs is crucial in addressing these challenges and ensuring that the rights of children with disabilities are realized through quality, accessible education.

3.4   Outcomes of Educational Interventions

Educational interventions in low- and middle-income countries (LMICs) have been shown to improve various outcomes for students with disabilities. This section explores the academic, social, and economic benefits of inclusive education, as well as the challenges in evaluating these outcomes.

- **Academic Outcomes:** Educational interventions, including the use of assistive technologies, specialized teacher training, and adapted learning materials, have shown positive impacts on literacy, numeracy, and overall academic performance among students with disabilities. Studies in countries like Uganda and India indicate that children with disabilities who participate in inclusive education programs demonstrate improved academic outcomes compared to their peers in segregated schools (Okech et al., 2021).
- **Social and Economic Outcomes**: Beyond academic achievements, inclusive education interventions have contributed to greater social integration and improved employment prospects for people with disabilities in LMICs. Students with disabilities who are integrated into mainstream schools are more likely to develop social skills, build friendships, and access future employment opportunities, leading to greater independence and societal participation (OECD, 2022).
- **Evaluation Methods**: The evaluation of outcomes in educational inclusion is often hampered by a lack of standardized frameworks. Many studies rely on small sample sizes and short-term assessments, limiting findings' generalizability and long-term insights. Greater emphasis on longitudinal studies and rigorous evaluation metrics is needed to accurately assess the impact of inclusive education programs (Mpu & Adu, 2021).

Table 3.2 provides a summary of the key outcomes of educational interventions for students with disabilities in low- and middle-income countries (LMICs). It highlights the academic, social, and economic benefits of inclusive education, as well as the challenges associated with evaluating these outcomes.

3.5   Gaps in Research

- **Underexplored Areas**: Key areas of research that remain underexplored include the intersectionality of disability and other social factors such as gender, ethnicity, and socioeconomic status. Longitudinal studies examining the long-term effects of inclusive education on students with disabilities are also lacking. Additionally, the non-academic impacts, such as improvements in quality of life and social integration, require more attention (Kelly et al., 2022). For instance, in some parts of South Asia, girls with disabilities face double discrimination based on both

Table 3.2 Outcomes of educational interventions for students with disabilities in low- and middle-income countries (LMICs)

Outcome Area	Description	Key Findings
Academic Outcomes	Impact on literacy, numeracy, and academic performance through assistive technologies and specialized teacher training	Students in inclusive education programs show improved academic performance compared to those in segregated schools
Social and Economic Outcomes	Contribution to social integration and future employment prospects	Inclusive education promotes social skills, friendships, and independence, leading to better employment opportunities
Evaluation Methods	• Challenges in assessing outcomes due to lack of standardized frameworks and short-term assessments	Need for longitudinal studies and rigorous evaluation metrics to accurately assess the impact of inclusive education programs

gender and disability, which further limits their access to education compared to their male counterparts.

- **Methodological Issues:** Methodological challenges in researching educational inclusion include the reliance on small sample sizes, the lack of standardized data collection tools, and the limited use of mixed-methods approaches. These issues hinder the development of robust evidence on the effectiveness of inclusive education interventions (Mpu & Adu, 2021). Small sample sizes and the absence of longitudinal studies contribute to a fragmented understanding of educational outcomes for students with disabilities, limiting the ability to develop universally applicable best practices.

- **Geographical Gaps:** The geographical gap in research on educational inclusion in low- and middle-income countries (LMICs) often highlights an uneven focus. Much of the research centers on Sub-Saharan Africa and South Asia, leaving regions like the Middle East and Latin America less explored. This geographical imbalance limits the global understanding of the effectiveness and challenges of educational inclusion across diverse regions. The emphasis on particular areas over others may stem from historical, socioeconomic, and political factors that affect the accessibility and quality of education in these regions. Research by the World Bank underscores these regional disparities, revealing that while Sub-Saharan Africa and South Asia often receive more focus, the Middle East and Latin America are significantly underrepresented in educational inclusion studies (World Bank, 2020). Furthermore, reports from organizations like UNICEF suggest that technological interventions, such as personalized learning tools, are frequently assessed in specific regions but lack comparative studies across different educational systems, particularly those in the Middle East and Latin America (UNICEF, 2019). Addressing this imbalance is crucial for understanding and improving educational inclusion globally. While Sub-Saharan Africa and South Asia have received substantial research attention, the Middle East and parts of Latin America remain underrepresented in inclusive education studies, potentially resulting in missed opportunities for global learning and application.

3.6 Recommendations for Future Studies

- **Policy Research**: Future research should focus on evidence-based policymaking, examining the effectiveness of various inclusive education policies and their scalability across different regions and contexts. Policymakers should be encouraged to invest in data collection and analysis to inform their decisions. Future studies should assess the success of inclusive education policies and investigate the processes through which these policies are implemented and how they can be adapted to meet the unique needs of local contexts in LMICs.
- **Innovative Practices**: The role of emerging technologies and innovative teaching methods, such as online learning platforms and digital assistive tools, should be studied to assess their potential for enhancing educational inclusion, particularly in remote and rural areas. Innovative practices, such as AI-powered assistive devices and remote learning platforms, could play a pivotal role in overcoming geographical and infrastructural challenges in rural areas.
- Stakeholder Involvement: It is essential to involve all stakeholders—students, families, teachers, and communities—in research on educational inclusion. Their perspectives are crucial for understanding inclusive education's challenges and opportunities and designing more effective interventions.

3.7 Conclusion

This chapter has explored the barriers to educational inclusion for people with disabilities in LMICs, the effectiveness of existing policies, and the outcomes of interventions. While significant progress has been made in aligning educational systems with international frameworks, substantial challenges remain. Addressing physical inaccessibility, social stigma, and economic constraints is essential for full inclusion. By prioritizing inclusive education, improving infrastructure, and fostering community involvement, LMICs can better integrate people with disabilities into educational systems, ultimately improving their social, economic, and academic outcomes. Fostering multi-sectoral collaboration and focusing on policy reform and community engagement will help create more inclusive and equitable educational environments for students with disabilities, enhancing their academic and social outcomes.

References

Eleweke, C. J. (1999). The need for mandatory legislations to enhance services to people with disabilities in Nigeria. *Disability & Society, 14*(2), 227–237. https://doi.org/10.1080/096875 99926299

Global Partnership for Education. (2018). *The challenges of implementing inclusive education policies in LMICs.* https://www.globalpartnership.org

Global Partnership for Education. (2020). *Challenges and solutions in inclusive education for children with disabilities.* https://www.globalpartnership.org

Hayes, A. M., & Bulat, J. (2017). *Disabilities inclusive education systems and policies guide for low- and middle-income countries.* RTI Press. https://www.ncbi.nlm.nih.gov/books/NBK554 622/ https://doi.org/10.3768/rtipress.2017.op.0043.1707

International Disability Alliance. (2021). *Global report on disability-inclusive education.* https:// www.internationaldisabilityalliance.org

Kelly, J., Mckenzie, J., Watermeyer, B., Vergunst, R., Karisa, A., & Samuels, C. (2022). We need to go back to our schools, and we need to make that change we wish to see': Empowering teachers for disability inclusion. *International Journal of Disability, Development and Education, 71*(4), 633–649. https://doi.org/10.1080/1034912X.2022.2141696

Mariga, L., McConkey, R., & Myezwa, H. (2014). *Inclusive education in low-income countries: A resource book for teacher educators, parent trainers, and community development workers.* Atlas Alliance and Disability Innovations Africa.

Mpu, Y., & Adu, E. O. (2021). The challenges of inclusive education and its implementation in schools: The South African perspective. *Perspectives in Education, 39*(2), 225–238. https://doi. org/10.38140/pie.v39i2.4583

OECD. (2022). *The social and economic rationale of inclusive education.* Organisation for Economic Co-operation and Development. https://www.oecd.org/content/dam/oecd/en/public ations/reports/2022/01/the-social-and-economic-rationale-of-inclusive-education_56b45b9c/ bff7a85d-en.pdf

Okech, J. B., Yuwono, I., & JumaAbdu, W. (2021). Implementation of inclusive education practices for children with disabilities and other special needs in Uganda. *Journal of Education and e-Learning Research, 8*(1), 97–102. https://www.researchgate.net/publication/349280444_Imp lementation_of_Inclusive_Education_Practices_for_Children_with_Disabilities_and_Other_ Special_Needs_in_Uganda. Accessed December 8 2024.

RTI International. (2022). *Disabilities inclusion guides for low- and middle-income countries.* https://www.rti.org

Sightsavers. (2021). *Inclusive education strategy.* Sightsavers. https://www.sightsavers.org/wp-con tent/uploads/2021/07/Sightsavers-Inclusive-Education-Strategy.pdf

UNESCO. (2019). *Monitoring inclusive education in Sub-Saharan Africa: Regional report.* https:// www.unesco.org

UNESCO. (2021). *Inclusion and education: All means all.* https://www.unesco.org

UNICEF. (2019). *Inclusive education: A critical component of the right to education.* United Nations Children's Fund. https://www.unicef.org

UNICEF. (2020). *Education and disability: Ensuring equity and inclusion for all children.* https:// www.unicef.org

United Nations. (2017). *The sustainable development goals report 2017.* United Nations. https:// unstats.un.org/sdgs/report/2017/Goal-04/

United Nations Development Programme. (2024). *Quality education: Goal 4.* United Nations Development Programme. Retrieved December 8, 2024, from https://www.undp.org/sustainable-dev elopment-goals/quality-education

World Bank. (2018). *Disability inclusion in education: Addressing social barriers to access.* https://
www.worldbank.org
World Bank. (2020). *Inclusive education: Achieving education for all by including those with
disabilities.* https://www.worldbank.org
World Health Organization (WHO) & World Bank. (2011). *World report on disability.* World Health
Organization. https://www.who.int/publications/i/item/9789240685215

Chapter 4
Employment and Disability in LMICs

Abstract This chapter explore the employment challenges and opportunities for individuals with disabilities in low- and middle-income countries (LMICs), exploring factors such as workforce participation, discrimination, and the efficacy of employment programs. It underscores the profound economic implications of disability-inclusive employment, highlighting its role in promoting social inclusion and economic stability. This chapter also identifies crucial research gaps, urging future exploration to better understand the intersections between disability, employment, and societal dynamics. While people with disabilities in LMICs face numerous barriers—ranging from physical inaccessibility and discriminatory attitudes to limited vocational training—employment remains a key driver of social integration. Moreover, inclusive employment supports the achievement of the Sustainable Development Goals (SDGs), particularly Goal 8, which advocates for inclusive and sustainable economic growth. This chapter presents a comprehensive analysis of these issues, with a call to action for more robust policies, research, and practices that can foster inclusive labor markets and improve outcomes for people with disabilities in LMICs.

4.1 Barriers to Employment

People with disabilities in low- and middle-income countries (LMICs) face a range of significant barriers to gaining employment, which are rooted in both systemic and societal challenges. These barriers limit access to the labor market and hinder the full participation of individuals with disabilities in the workforce, contributing to high rates of unemployment and underemployment. Addressing these barriers is essential for creating more inclusive and equitable employment opportunities for people with disabilities.

© The Author(s), under exclusive license to Springer Nature Singapore Pte Ltd. 2025   33
A. Al Shami and A. J. Nashwan, *Global Health and Disability*,
SpringerBriefs in Modern Perspectives on Disability Research,
https://doi.org/10.1007/978-981-96-4956-3_4

- **Systemic Barriers**

Persons with disabilities in LMICs face significant structural challenges that impede their access to the labor market. One of the most prominent barriers is inaccessible infrastructure, including the lack of accessible workplaces, transportation, and accommodations for people with mobility impairments. Many workspaces, particularly in low-resource settings, do not have ramps, elevators, or accessible restrooms, making it difficult for people with disabilities to navigate their environments (Chetty, 2024).

In addition to these physical barriers, the lack of effective enforcement of disability-inclusive policies is another systemic challenge. Although many LMICs have laws designed to promote the employment of people with disabilities, they are often inadequately enforced due to weak governance structures and limited monitoring. For example, a review of employment challenges in South Asia and Africa highlighted the absence of tailored interventions for persons with disabilities, particularly the lack of enforcement of policies that would ensure equal access to employment (Morwane et al., 2021). Without the necessary legal frameworks and enforcement, the potential for persons with disabilities to access the labor market remains limited.

Further complicating matters is the limited availability of vocational training and education programs that are adapted to the specific needs of people with disabilities. Vocational training centers in many LMICs do not offer the necessary resources to accommodate diverse disabilities, preventing people from acquiring the necessary skills to succeed in the workforce.

- **Discrimination and Stigma**

Discrimination and stigma are deeply ingrained societal challenges that act as significant barriers to employment for people with disabilities in LMICs. Social stigma against disability often manifests as employers' negative attitudes toward hiring individuals with disabilities, driven by misconceptions that they are less capable or require excessive support. A study on employment challenges in South Africa found that discriminatory attitudes were particularly prevalent in small and medium-sized enterprises (SMEs), where employers often view hiring people with disabilities as an additional burden (McGrath et al., 2010).

This societal stigma is compounded by mental health-related stigma, which also influences employment opportunities for individuals with disabilities. Mental health stigma, pervasive at structural, societal, and individual levels, significantly exacerbates challenges faced by vulnerable groups, including people with disabilities. This stigma, influenced by socio-cultural and systemic factors, limits access to employment and leads to unfavorable outcomes such as poor adherence to treatment and reduced opportunities for social integration (Vaishnav et al., 2023). Despite the implementation of some policy changes in LMICs, such as in Kenya, negative attitudes toward hiring individuals with disabilities persist, particularly in the context of mental health issues (Barbareschi et al., 2021). These entrenched discriminatory practices contribute to the hostile work environment and prevent individuals from fully participating in the workforce (Morwane et al., 2021).

- **Attitudinal Barriers**

Attitudinal barriers, rooted in deeply held cultural and societal beliefs, are also a significant factor in the exclusion of persons with disabilities from the workforce. In many LMICs, people with disabilities are perceived as unable to contribute meaningfully to the workforce. These attitudes, shaped by longstanding cultural stigmas, lead to a lack of awareness about the potential of individuals with disabilities to succeed in competitive employment. In some cases, even family members of individuals with disabilities hold limiting beliefs, preventing them from encouraging the pursuit of educational or vocational opportunities (Morwane et al., 2021).

4.2 Facilitators of Employment

While significant barriers exist, there are also numerous factors that can enhance employment outcomes for people with disabilities in low- and middle-income countries (LMICs). Various policies, programs, and practices have proven effective in addressing challenges and creating more inclusive employment environments. This section explores the key facilitators, focusing on supportive policies, vocational training, and workplace accommodations, which can help individuals with disabilities gain meaningful employment and thrive in the workforce.

- **Supportive Policies and Programs**

Despite the challenges, several programs and policies have shown promise in improving employment outcomes for persons with disabilities in LMICs. One of the most effective models has been the Individual Placement and Support (IPS) program, which emphasizes placing individuals with disabilities into competitive employment while providing ongoing support such as job coaching and mental health services. Studies have shown that IPS leads to better employment outcomes than traditional sheltered employment models (Chen & Lal, 2020; Steffens & Felix, 2022).

- **Vocational Training and Education**

Vocational training is essential for increasing the employability of persons with disabilities in LMICs. Training programs that focus on marketable skills—such as information technology, carpentry, or administrative tasks—are crucial in preparing individuals for competitive jobs. However, vocational training programs need to be tailored to meet the needs of people with different types of disabilities, whether physical, intellectual, or mental health related.

All included studies reported positive impacts on livelihood outcomes. However, due to variation between studies, it is difficult to draw firm conclusions about what works, for whom, and how (Hunt et al., 2022). Most studies focused on improving access to the workplace, with interventions such as involving people without disabilities in programs aimed at improving their social attitudes toward working with people with disabilities, providing wheelchairs for those with mobility impairments, and placing individuals with disabilities in supported employment positions.

Studies have examined various approaches, including vocational training programs, a "motivation to work" program, community-based rehabilitation, and social skills training. All of these approaches showed positive impacts on livelihood outcomes, including finding employment, acquiring skills for the workplace, and gaining social skills needed for work (Hunt et al., 2022).

Furthermore, these programs have led to improved outcomes for people with disabilities in terms of acquiring skills for the workplace, gaining access to the job market, securing employment in both formal and informal sectors, and accessing social protection measures. Future research should focus on evaluating these approaches with more rigorous study designs, which would contribute to a firmer evidence base and inform the delivery of interventions at scale.

Partnerships between governments, NGOs, and private organizations can ensure that these programs are designed inclusively and provide the necessary support for individuals to succeed (Chetty, 2024; Steffens & Felix, 2022).

- **Workplace Accommodations**

In order for persons with disabilities to thrive in the workforce, workplaces need to provide reasonable accommodations. These accommodations can range from physical adaptations, such as ramps or accessible workstations, to adjustments in job responsibilities, such as offering flexible hours for individuals with psychiatric disabilities who may need more time for self-care. Educating employers about the importance and feasibility of these accommodations is critical. Many employers are unaware of the simple changes that can significantly enhance productivity and inclusivity (Chetty, 2024; Felix, 2021).

To provide a clearer overview of these key barriers and facilitators, Table 4.1 summarizes the main factors, as discussed in the previous sections. It offers a concise comparison between the barriers and the actions or conditions that can facilitate better employment outcomes for people with disabilities in LMICs.

4.3   Economic Implications

The economic benefits of employing persons with disabilities extend beyond the individual level. Research has shown that inclusive employment policies can lead to broader economic growth, particularly in LMICs. By tapping into a previously underutilized labor pool, countries can increase their overall productivity and reduce the economic burden of disability-related poverty. Furthermore, as persons with disabilities achieve greater economic independence, they contribute to tax revenues, reduce reliance on government welfare programs, and become active consumers in the economy (Steffens, 2021).

Table 4.1 Barriers and facilitators to employment for people with disabilities in LMICs

Category	Barriers	Facilitators
Systemic Barriers	Inaccessible infrastructure (e.g., workplaces, transportation)	Supportive policies (e.g., Individual Placement and Support program)
Discrimination & Stigma	Negative attitudes toward hiring people with disabilities	Awareness campaigns to reduce stigma and discrimination
Attitudinal Barriers	Societal and cultural beliefs about the capabilities of individuals with disabilities	Vocational training tailored to the needs of individuals with disabilities
Workplace Accommodations	Lack of reasonable accommodations (e.g., ramps, flexible working hours)	Provision of workplace accommodations (e.g., accessible workstations, job coaching)
Vocational Training	Limited access to vocational training programs for people with disabilities	Effective vocational training programs focusing on marketable skills (IT, carpentry)

In South Africa, the importance of economic empowerment for people with disabilities has been highlighted in national policies and recent government initiatives. President Cyril Ramaphosa, in his keynote address at the Summit on Economic Empowerment of Persons with Disabilities in 2022, emphasized the need for people with disabilities to be actively involved in the creation and implementation of economic policies. The government aims to break down barriers that prevent their full participation in the economy and has committed to ensuring equal access to land, capital, infrastructure, and decent work. This includes specific programs targeting self-employment, entrepreneurship, and cooperatives for people with disabilities, alongside efforts to strengthen vocational training and career advancement opportunities (SANews, 2022).

Furthermore, the White Paper on the Rights of Persons with Disabilities outlines strategic measures to reduce economic vulnerability for people with disabilities, focusing on removing barriers to access and promoting their empowerment. One of the key goals is to unlock human capital by facilitating access to economic opportunities, which includes improving education and employment conditions for people with disabilities (South Africa, 2016).

These initiatives aim to promote a more inclusive society by addressing economic inequalities and empowering individuals with disabilities through comprehensive policy changes and targeted programs.

A report from the International Labour Organization (ILO) estimated that increasing employment for people with disabilities could reduce disability-related welfare costs by up to 30% in low-income countries (Ananian & Dellaferrera, 2024).

Figure 4.1 illustrates the positive economic outcomes associated with disability-inclusive employment in low- and middle-income countries (LMICs).

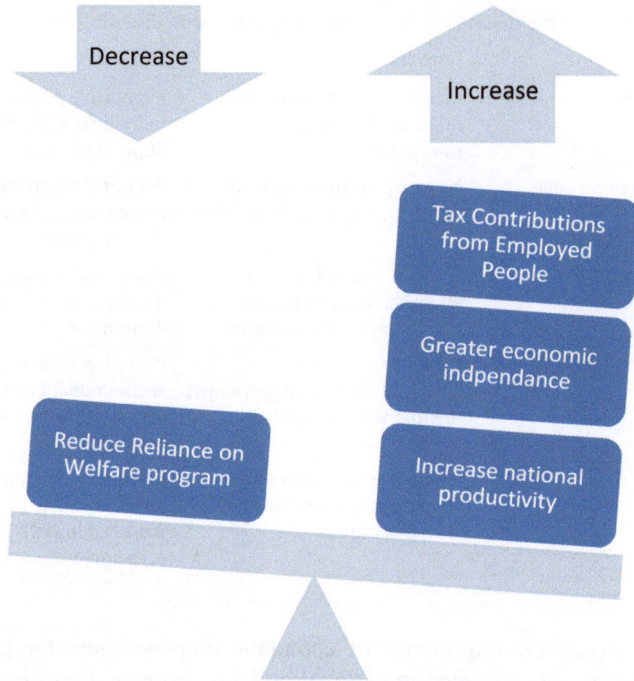

Fig. 4.1 Economic impact of disability-inclusive employment in LMICs

4.4 Research Gaps and Recommendations

Despite progress, there remain substantial gaps in the literature on disability-inclusive employment in LMICs. Much of the research focuses on a small subset of countries, and there is a need for more data from diverse regions. Research should explore the long-term outcomes of supported employment programs and how they can be scaled to meet the needs of different populations.

In particular, more research is needed on the intersectionality of disability and gender, as women with disabilities face additional challenges in accessing employment, such as gender-based discrimination and societal expectations regarding caregiving. Future studies should examine how policies can address these compounded barriers (Steffens, 2021).

Finally, future research should focus on developing contextualized models for disability-inclusive employment that consider the cultural, economic, and political environments of LMICs. This would help ensure that programs and policies are relevant and effective in each specific context (Morwane et al., 2021).

4.5 Conclusion

Addressing the employment challenges faced by persons with disabilities in low- and middle-income countries (LMICs) requires a multifaceted approach that includes systemic policy reforms, awareness campaigns, and tailored support programs. Governments, employers, and civil society organizations must collaborate to create an inclusive labor market that offers opportunities for all individuals, regardless of their abilities. Employment is not just an economic necessity but also a fundamental element of social inclusion and empowerment for persons with disabilities. By overcoming existing barriers and providing appropriate support, LMICs can help individuals with disabilities achieve economic independence, enhance their quality of life, and contribute to sustainable development. To truly empower individuals with disabilities, LMICs must prioritize comprehensive policy reforms, invest in vocational training, and build a robust infrastructure that supports all workers, regardless of their abilities.

References

Ananian, S., & Dellaferrera, G. (2024). *A study on the employment and wage outcomes of people with disabilities* (ILO Working Paper 124). https://doi.org/10.54394/YRCN8597

Barbareschi, G., Carew, M. T., Johnson, E. A., Kopi, N., & Holloway, C. (2021). "When they see a wheelchair, they've not even seen me"—Factors shaping the experience of disability stigma and discrimination in Kenya. *International Journal of Environmental Research and Public Health, 18*(8), 4272. https://doi.org/10.3390/ijerph18084272

Chen, N., & Lal, S. (2020). Stakeholder perspectives on IPS for employment: A scoping review. *Canadian Journal of Occupational Therapy, 87*(4), 307–318. https://doi.org/10.1177/000841 7420946611

Chetty, L. (2024). Factors that influence the employment of people with disabilities from low- to medium-income countries. *IOSR Journal of Nursing and Health Science (IOSR-JNHS), 13*(3), 19–27. https://doi.org/10.9790/1959-1303051927

Felix, L. (2021). *Evidence brief: What is the evidence of successful interventions that increase employment and livelihood participation for people with psychosocial disability?* Disability Evidence Portal.

Hunt, X., Saran, A., Banks, L. M., White, H., & Kuper, H. (2022). Effectiveness of interventions for improving livelihood outcomes for people with disabilities in low- and middle-income countries: A systematic review. *Campbell Systematic Reviews, 18*, e1257. https://doi.org/10.1002/cl2.1257

McGrath, L., Jones, R. S., & Hastings, R. P. (2010). Outcomes of anti-bullying intervention for adults with intellectual disabilities. *Research in Developmental Disabilities, 31*(2), 376–380. https://doi.org/10.1016/j.ridd.2009.10.006

Morwane, R. E., Dada, S., & Bornman, J. (2021). Barriers to and facilitators of employment of persons with disabilities in low- and middle-income countries: A scoping review. *African Journal of Disability, 10*, a833. https://doi.org/10.4102/ajod.v10i0.833

SANews. (2022, December 7). *Include people with disabilities in the implementation of economic development policies*. South African Government News Agency. https://www.sanews.gov.za/south-africa/include-people-disabilities-implementation-economic-development-policies

South Africa. (2016, March 23). *White paper on the rights of persons with disabilities* (Government Notice No. 230). Government Printing Works. https://www.gov.za/sites/default/files/gcis_docu ment/201603/39792gon230.pdf

Steffens, L. (2021). *Evidence brief: What is the impact of inclusive employment for persons with disabilities?* Disability Evidence Portal. https://disabilityevidence.org/

Steffens, L., & Felix, L. (2022). *Evidence brief: What is the current evidence around employment interventions that specifically focus on people with intellectual and developmental disabilities.* Disability Evidence Portal.

Vaishnav, M., Javed, A., Gupta, S., Kumar, V., Vaishnav, P., Kumar, A., Salih, H., Bernardo, N. G., Levounis, P., NG, B., Alkhoori, S., Luguercho, C., Soghoyan, A., Moore, E., Lakra, V., Aigner, M., Wancata, J., Ismayilova, J., Azizul Islam, M., … Ashurov. (2023). Stigma towards mental illness in Asian nations and low-and-middle-income countries, and comparison with high-income countries: A literature review and practice implications. *Indian Journal of Psychiatry, 65*(10), 995–1011.

Chapter 5
Socio-Cultural Perceptions of Disability in LMICs

Abstract This chapter examines the socio-cultural dimensions of disability in Low-and Middle-Income Countries (LMICs), focusing on cultural beliefs, social norms, religious practices, and the pervasive stigma surrounding disability. It explores how these factors shape the experiences and inclusion of individuals with disabilities in LMICs, often exacerbating social exclusion and marginalization. This chapter highlights the role of cultural narratives and religious interpretations in shaping societal attitudes and policies, the impact of stigma and discrimination, and the challenges faced by individuals with disabilities and their families. It also explores how these socio-cultural perceptions intersect with other social categories such as gender, age, and socioeconomic status, deepening the marginalization of some groups. Drawing on recent studies, this chapter presents strategies for addressing these challenges, including community engagement, policy interventions, and leveraging religious and cultural leadership. It concludes with a call for global cooperation and the exchange of best practices to foster inclusive societies that respect the dignity and rights of people with disabilities.

5.1 Understanding Cultural Beliefs and Norms

Cultural beliefs profoundly influence the perception of disability in LMICs. In many traditional societies, disability is often viewed through fatalistic lenses, being associated with divine punishment, parental sins, or a test of faith (Holzer et al., 1999). Such beliefs can discourage families from seeking medical or educational interventions, as they may be seen as defying divine will.

Families often play a central role in shaping the experience of individuals with disabilities. However, the degree of support can vary significantly. While some families provide strong emotional and material backing, others may internalize stigma, further marginalizing affected individuals. For example, families from rural areas or with lower socioeconomic status may experience heightened shame or reluctance to seek support due to perceived community judgment. Community attitudes, including those that ostracize or pity individuals with disabilities, can perpetuate this cycle of exclusion (Saad & Borowska-Beszta, 2019).

These cultural norms are not homogeneous. Regional variations within LMICs reflect differences in history, socioeconomic conditions, and exposure to modern disability rights frameworks. In urban areas, where there may be more exposure to global disability rights movements, individuals with disabilities may have more access to inclusive services, whereas in rural areas, traditional views may dominate, hindering progress. Understanding these nuances is critical to designing culturally sensitive interventions.

5.2   Religious Influences on Disability Perception

Religion is a double-edged sword in disability discourse within LMICs. On one hand, Islamic teachings, for instance, advocate for compassion and inclusivity, emphasizing the dignity of individuals with disabilities. Families often draw strength from religious principles, finding solace in caregiving (Al-Aoufi et al., 2012). On the other hand, interpretations that frame disabilities as divine tests or misfortunes can reinforce stigma.

Engaging religious leaders to promote positive narratives can have transformative effects. Leaders who emphasize inclusion and equality can reshape community attitudes, making religious institutions critical allies in disability advocacy (Khayat et al., 2024). For instance, Islamic teachings highlight the importance of caring for those with disabilities as an act of kindness, which can be used as a framework to reduce stigma. Conversely, charity-focused approaches that overlook empowerment perpetuate dependency and hinder long-term inclusion.

5.3   Stigma and Discrimination

Stigma remains one of the most significant barriers to inclusion for individuals with disabilities. It manifests in social exclusion, limited access to services, and discriminatory practices in education, employment, and healthcare. This stigma often extends to families, creating cycles of isolation and economic hardship. Stigma can also be compounded by traditional beliefs in the "curse" of disability, which can lead to the marginalization of the entire family, not just the individual with a disability.

The intersectionality of stigma compounds its impact. Women with disabilities, for example, often face dual discrimination based on gender and disability. Similarly, poverty exacerbates barriers to accessing resources and support (Ilyas et al., 2021). The challenges faced by rural women with disabilities may be further compounded by their roles as caregivers for other family members, which limits their opportunities for education and employment.

Systemic issues, such as weak policy enforcement and limited funding, further entrench discrimination. Without robust legal protections and resources to implement them, individuals with disabilities remain marginalized (World Health Organization, 2018). These systemic issues often stem from a lack of disability-inclusive policies and inadequate awareness among policymakers, which leads to gaps in implementation and enforcement.

5.4 Policy and Advocacy: Addressing Socio-Cultural Barriers

Disability-inclusive policies in LMICs have made progress but still face significant gaps. Many countries have ratified the United Nations Convention on the Rights of Persons with Disabilities (CRPD), signaling their commitment to inclusion. However, translating these commitments into actionable policies is challenging due to weak enforcement mechanisms, limited inter-agency coordination, and insufficient funding (DESA, 2007).

Innovative advocacy models, such as grassroots movements and digital platforms, are helping to bridge these gaps. Community-based approaches have shown promise in reducing stigma and promoting inclusion. Programs that involve local leaders, families, and individuals with disabilities in awareness campaigns and service delivery have proven effective in changing attitudes. For example, youth-led advocacy movements that leverage social media can amplify disability inclusion messages, creating ripple effects across communities.

Media and education systems are underutilized tools in this effort. Inclusive curricula and anti-stigma training for educators can foster acceptance from an early age. Media campaigns that highlight the achievements and potential of individuals with disabilities can also shift public perceptions. Governments and NGOs should partner to develop targeted educational campaigns in schools and local media, showcasing role models and the capabilities of individuals with disabilities.

5.5 Case Studies and Best Practices

Successful initiatives in LMICs demonstrate that change is possible. For instance, the UAE's national policy for empowering individuals with disabilities focuses on inclusive education, employment opportunities, and community integration. Similarly, Qatar's Vision 2030 includes comprehensive strategies for disability inclusion, providing models that other LMICs can adapt (Al Hadad, 2023; Medabesh et al., 2024).

Community-based rehabilitation programs in rural regions of LMICs have also achieved significant progress. These programs emphasize local leadership, participatory planning, and the integration of services, offering a blueprint for scalable solutions.

- **South Africa's Integrated Disability Services:** South Africa has implemented an integrated approach to disability services that incorporates both health and social services, emphasizing early intervention and the importance of family support. One such program, the "Disability and Rehabilitation Policy," provides a coordinated response to the needs of individuals with disabilities, ensuring that services such as mobility aids, healthcare, and education are accessible. The approach has shown positive impacts on the social inclusion of individuals with disabilities, as well as on their access to essential services (Samuels et al., 2012).
- **Kenya's Disability-Inclusive Employment Policies:** In Kenya, national legislation mandating the employment of individuals with disabilities has led to the establishment of various inclusive workplaces. For example, the Kenya National Council for Persons with Disabilities (NCPWD) collaborates with both public and private sector employers to create job opportunities, ensuring workplace adaptations and inclusive hiring practices. This initiative has improved the livelihoods of people with disabilities, enhancing their economic independence and social integration (Mastercard Foundation, 2023)

5.6   Future Directions

Addressing the socio-cultural dimensions of disability requires a multifaceted approach. Research gaps, particularly on the intersectionality of stigma and systemic barriers, must be addressed. Comprehensive data collection and disability registries are essential for designing targeted interventions and monitoring progress (World Health Organization, 2018).

Policymakers should focus on inclusive education, robust legal protections, and community engagement. Innovative approaches, such as leveraging digital platforms for awareness and service delivery, can also play a pivotal role. Additionally, strengthening the capacity of local organizations and community leaders to advocate for disability rights can ensure sustainability and long-term impact.

5.7   Conclusion

The socio-cultural landscape of disability in LMICs presents both challenges and opportunities. By addressing cultural beliefs, religious narratives, and systemic barriers, societies can foster greater inclusion and equality. Community-driven initiatives, informed by cultural insights and supported by strong policy frameworks, hold the key to transforming attitudes and improving the quality of life for individuals with disabilities. As the global community continues to embrace disability inclusion, it is essential to prioritize cultural sensitivity and local context in designing solutions that are sustainable and effective.

References

Al Hadad, A. H. (2023). *Inclusion of people with disability in sport: A case study of Qatar*. Hamad Bin Khalifa University.

Al-Aoufi, H., Al-Zyoud, N., & Shahminan, N. (2012). Islam and the cultural conceptualisation of disability. *International Journal of Adolescence and Youth, 17*(4), 205–219.

Holzer, B., Vreede, A., & Weigt, G. (Eds.). (1999). *Disability in different cultures: Reflections on local concept*. Transcript Verlag.

Ilyas, M., Siddiqui, A. A., Afroze, E., Al-Enizy, A. S., & Alam, M. K. (2021). Developmental disabilities in the Arab World. In *Handbook of healthcare in the Arab World* (pp. 2177–2195). Springer.

Khayat, A. M., Alshareef, B. G., Alharbi, S. F., AlZahrani, M. M., Alshangity, B. A., & Tashkandi, N. F. (2024). Consanguineous marriage and its association with genetic disorders in Saudi Arabia: A review. *Cureus, 16*(2), e53888.

Mastercard Foundation. (2023). *Kenya full report*. https://mastercardfdn.org/wp-content/uploads/2023/02/Kenya-Full-Report.pdf

Medabesh, A. M., Malik, N. N., Shafi, M., & Rashid, J. (2024). Employment scenario for people with disabilities (PWDs) in Saudi Arabia: Challenges and opportunities. *Journal of Disability Research, 3*(7), 20240090.

Saad, M. A. E., & Borowska-Beszta, B. (2019). Disability in the Arab World: A comparative analysis within culture. *International Journal of Psycho-Educational Sciences, 8*(2), 29–47.

Samuels, A., Slemming, W., & Balton, S. (2012). Early childhood intervention in South Africa in relation to the developmental systems model. *Infants & Young Children, 25*, 334–345. https://doi.org/10.1097/IYC.0b013e3182673e12

United Nations Department of Economic and Social Affairs (DESA). (2007). *Division of Social Policy and Development (DSPD), in collaboration with UNESCO and UN-HABITAT*. United Nations.

World Health Organization. (2018). *Disability and health in the Eastern Mediterranean region*.

Chapter 6
Disability Rights and Policy in LMICs

Abstract This chapter explores the state of disability rights and policies in low- and middle-income countries (LMICs), with particular attention to the implementation of international conventions like the United Nations Convention on the Rights of Persons with Disabilities (UNCRPD). By examining national legal frameworks, the role of advocacy groups, and the impact of Disabled People's Organizations (DPOs), this chapter highlights both the successes and challenges in advancing disability rights. Key barriers to the implementation of disability policies include resource limitations, political will, and societal stigma, which often lead to exclusion in areas such as education, employment, and healthcare. Despite these challenges, successful examples of disability-inclusive policies in regions like Latin America offer valuable lessons for improving accessibility and social participation. This chapter concludes with a call for stronger policy integration, particularly within broader development strategies, and urges increased research to address the intersectional challenges faced by persons with disabilities in LMICs. Recommendations include enhancing accessibility, strengthening cross-sector collaboration, and integrating disability inclusion into national and global agendas, such as the Sustainable Development Goals (SDGs) and climate change adaptation.

6.1 Overview

The inclusion of persons with disabilities within national and international policies remains a critical issue in LMICs, where socioeconomic factors, cultural barriers, and limited infrastructure hinder the realization of their rights. International agreements, such as the UNCRPD, call for comprehensive policies to ensure equal opportunities, non-discrimination, and full participation of persons with disabilities in society. However, LMICs face substantial challenges in implementing these commitments due to financial constraints, lack of political will, and infrastructural barriers. Moreover, there is often a lack of awareness about the scope of disability inclusion, further exacerbating the challenges in policy enforcement.

A. Al Shami and A. J. Nashwan, *Global Health and Disability*,
SpringerBriefs in Modern Perspectives on Disability Research,
https://doi.org/10.1007/978-981-96-4956-3_6

A critical element in overcoming these barriers is addressing the intersectionality of disability with other forms of social exclusion, such as gender, age, and socioeconomic status. Women and children with disabilities in LMICs often face compounded challenges that must be considered in policy design.

6.2 International Conventions and Frameworks

The UNCRPD, adopted in 2006, plays a central role in shaping global disability rights. It promotes a paradigm shift from seeing disability as a medical condition to viewing it as a social issue, focusing on human rights and the removal of barriers. The Sustainable Development Goals (SDGs), adopted in 2015, further reinforce the need for disability inclusion, with several goals directly or indirectly addressing the challenges faced by persons with disabilities (The United Nations, 2015). Despite these global frameworks, LMICs often struggle with the translation of these policies into actionable outcomes on the ground due to various factors including lack of resources and political attention. The implementation gap in LMICs remains a key challenge in translating international agreements into local solutions, often due to limited governmental capacity or conflicting policy priorities.

Additionally, regional variations in policy approaches can offer valuable insights. For instance, in Latin America, the emphasis on government-driven initiatives has led to stronger policies in the region, whereas in Africa, grassroots mobilization has proven effective in some countries, as seen with organizations such as the Kenya Society for the Blind.

6.3 National Legal Frameworks in LMICs

While many LMICs have enacted laws aimed at improving the rights of persons with disabilities, the implementation and enforcement of these laws remain limited. In India, for example, the Rights of Persons with Disabilities Act, 2016, emphasizes the need for accessibility and equal opportunity, but challenges persist in its implementation, particularly in rural areas (Math et al., 2019). In many African nations, disability laws exist but are often poorly enforced due to lack of funding, political will, and awareness among policymakers (Percy, 2018). There is also the issue of conflicting laws or lack of coordination between disability policies and other developmental policies, making it difficult to create a cohesive strategy for inclusion . Furthermore, the lack of intersectionality in policy approaches often leads to the marginalization of groups within the disability community, such as women, children, and those in rural or conflict-affected areas.

Some countries face additional challenges in policy implementation at local levels, where national laws often fail to translate into effective action due to limited local government capacity or resources. The lack of disability inclusion in local development strategies exacerbates this issue.

6.4 Barriers to Implementation of Disability Rights

LMICs face multiple barriers to the full implementation of disability rights. Socioeconomic barriers are perhaps the most significant, as persons with disabilities in these countries are often excluded from education, healthcare, and employment opportunities due to poverty and lack of accessible services. Structural barriers, including inaccessible transportation, buildings, and healthcare facilities, exacerbate the situation. Furthermore, cultural and societal stigma toward disability often results in marginalization and exclusion, making it difficult for persons with disabilities to participate fully in society (Khan et al., 2018).

Additionally, in several countries like Kenya, the lack of inclusive infrastructure and transportation has been identified as a major barrier. The Kenya Society for the Blind has been actively advocating for better access to public spaces and transportation systems for people with disabilities (Nyaura & Ngugi, 2019). These efforts are vital in addressing the systemic barriers that prevent full participation in society. Inadequate disability data and a lack of comprehensive disability inclusion frameworks at the local government level further hinder the identification and rectification of such barriers.

6.5 The Role of Advocacy Groups and Disabled People's Organizations (DPOs)

Advocacy groups, particularly Disabled People's Organizations (DPOs), have played a crucial role in advancing disability rights in LMICs. These organizations raise awareness, influence policy, and advocate for the inclusion of persons with disabilities in national development agendas (Grills et al., 2020). Successful advocacy efforts, such as those in East Africa and South Asia, have demonstrated the power of local DPOs in driving policy changes and improving access to services. However, DPOs often face challenges such as limited financial resources, political pushback, and the marginalization of their voices in policymaking processes (Young & Reeve, 2016). Nevertheless, these organizations remain key players in advocating for inclusive policies and building social support networks for persons with disabilities. The growing prominence of DPOs in the digital space has also provided new opportunities for advocacy and networking, albeit with challenges related to access and digital literacy.

6.6   Advancing Disability Rights: Effective Policies and Approaches

Some countries in LMICs have successfully implemented disability-inclusive policies. For example, several Latin American countries have introduced programs that promote the employment of persons with disabilities and provide financial assistance for disability-related healthcare needs (World Bank, 2021). These policies have had significant positive impacts on improving access to education, employment, and healthcare services. Additionally, there is growing recognition of the need to incorporate disability rights in broader development policies, particularly those related to social protection, poverty reduction, and healthcare.

Recommendations for advancing disability rights include improving accessibility in public services, providing financial incentives for businesses that employ persons with disabilities, and ensuring that educational institutions are inclusive. Governments should also work with local DPOs to implement programs that address the unique needs of persons with disabilities in areas such as healthcare, transportation, and housing. The need for greater cross-sector collaboration, particularly in health, education, and employment, has emerged as a critical strategy for strengthening disability inclusion policies.

6.7   Policy Gaps and Future Directions

Despite progress, gaps remain in disability-inclusive policies in LMICs. The literature points to a lack of comprehensive data on disability and an absence of specific research on the intersection of disability and climate change (Saran et al., 2020). Furthermore, disability policies are often not integrated into national development strategies, resulting in fragmented approaches that fail to address the root causes of exclusion (Lord et al., 2010). To fill these gaps, future policy research should focus on improving data collection and research on the barriers faced by persons with disabilities, particularly in rural and marginalized communities. It is also essential to integrate disability considerations into climate change adaptation policies and the growing digital economy. Emerging areas such as disability and digital inclusion, as well as the role of disability in humanitarian contexts, also require immediate attention in policy development.

Additionally, the role of international aid organizations and NGOs in driving policy change must not be overlooked. Many NGOs are critical in advocating for disability rights and providing services in areas where governments are unable to reach. These organizations can help bridge gaps in policy implementation and provide essential services to persons with disabilities.

6.8 Conclusion

The effective implementation of disability rights in LMICs is critical for ensuring the inclusion of persons with disabilities in society. While there are international conventions and national policies aimed at advancing these rights, challenges related to resource limitations, political will, and cultural attitudes hinder progress. However, through the active involvement of DPOs, successful policy examples, and increased attention to the barriers faced by persons with disabilities, there is potential for significant improvements. Future efforts must focus on creating inclusive policies that address the needs of persons with disabilities across various sectors, from education and healthcare to employment and climate change adaptation. The integration of disability considerations into broader global challenges, such as the SDGs, climate change, and technological advancements, will also play a key role in shaping a more inclusive future for persons with disabilities.

References

Grills, N. J., Hoq, M., Wong, C. P., Allah, K., Singh, L., Soji, F., & Murthy, G. S. (2020). Disabled people's organisations increase access to services and improve well-being: Evidence from a cluster randomized trial in North India. *BMC Public Health, 20*, 145. https://doi.org/10.1186/s12889-020-8192-0

Khan, F., Owolabi, M. O., Amatya, B., Hamzat, T. K., Ogunniyi, A., Oshinowo, H., Elmalik, A., & Galea, M. P. (2018). Challenges and barriers for implementation of the World Health Organization global disability action plan in low-and middle-income countries. *Journal of Rehabilitation Medicine (Stiftelsen Rehabiliteringsinformation), 50*(4), 367–376. https://doi.org/10.2340/16501977-2276

Lord, J., Posarac, A., Nicoli, M., Peffley, K., McClain-Nhlapo, C., & Keogh, M. (2010). *Disability and international cooperation and development: A review of policies and practices.* World Bank.

Math, S. B., Gowda, G. S., Basavaraju, V., Manjunatha, N., Kumar, C. N., Philip, S., & Gowda, M. (2019). The rights of persons with disability act, 2016: Challenges and opportunities. *Indian Journal of Psychiatry, 61*(Suppl 4), S809–S815. https://doi.org/10.4103/psychiatry.IndianJPsychiatry_105_19

Nyaura, J. E., & Ngugi, M. N. (2019). Accessing public transportation policies for persons living with disabilities in Kenya. *People: International Journal of Social Sciences, 5*(2), 801–817. https://doi.org/10.20319/pijss.2019.52.801817

Percy, S. L. (2018). *Disability, civil rights, and public policy: The politics of implementation.* University of Alabama Press.

Saran, A., White, H., & Kuper, H. (2020). Evidence and gap map of studies assessing the effectiveness of interventions for people with disabilities in low-and middle-income countries. *Campbell Systematic Reviews, 16*(1), e1070.

The United Nations. (2015). *Sustainable Development Goals (SDGs).* United Nations. Available at https://sdgs.un.org/goals

World Bank. (2021). *Disability inclusion in Latin America and the Caribbean: Easy read version.*
    https://thedocs.worldbank.org/en/doc/29c1baaa285d50c71ea1efeb259248ff-0370062021/ori
    ginal/Disability-Inclusion-in-Latin-America-and-the-Caribbean-Easy-Read-Version.pdf
Young, R., & Reeve, M. (2016). The functions of Disabled People's Organisations (DPOs) in low
    and middle-income countries: A literature review. *Disability, CBR & Inclusive Development,
    27*, 45. https://doi.org/10.5463/dcid.v27i3.539

Chapter 7
Innovations and Future Directions in Disability Research and Practice

Abstract This chapter provides a forward-looking review of emerging research and innovative practices in disability inclusion within low- and middle-income countries (LMICs). It explores technological advancements, innovative care models, and policy interventions, highlighting their impact on enhancing the lives of individuals with disabilities. This chapter concludes by proposing a research agenda to address existing gaps and advance disability inclusion efforts.

7.1 Overview

Disability inclusion has gained momentum globally, with increasing recognition of its critical importance in achieving sustainable development goals (SDGs). In LMICs, the challenges are multifaceted, including limited resources, infrastructural barriers, and cultural stigmas. Despite these hurdles, innovative solutions are emerging, ranging from technological advancements to inclusive policy frameworks, shaping a more equitable future for individuals with disabilities. This chapter also integrates recent findings from studies examining interventions aimed at improving social inclusion for people with disabilities in LMICs, which highlight the significant positive effects of various interventions (Saran et al., 2023). However, despite these advancements, the implementation of these interventions remains uneven, often hindered by financial and infrastructural limitations.

7.2 Technological Advancements

7.2.1 Assistive Technologies

The advent of affordable and adaptable assistive technologies has transformed disability inclusion. Devices such as low-cost prosthetics, mobility aids, and digital assistive solutions have made significant strides in improving accessibility. For instance, the introduction of 3D-printed prosthetics has reduced production costs, enabling broader access in resource-constrained settings (Goshe & Kassegne, 2022). Additionally, open-source technologies have gained traction, enabling local communities to develop affordable, customizable assistive devices tailored to their needs, making disability inclusion more sustainable in resource-limited settings (Chalkiadakis et al., 2024). These technologies have also shown promise in addressing accessibility gaps in both rural and urban settings, offering opportunities for scalable solutions.

7.2.2 Digital Innovations

Mobile health (mHealth) platforms and telehealth services have bridged geographical and financial gaps in healthcare delivery (Anawade et al., 2024; Haleem et al., 2021). AI technologies can improve access to information, education, and employment opportunities, thereby transforming lives and fostering a more inclusive world (UNRIC, 2024). **AI-powered applications**, such as speech-to-text converters and visual navigation tools, offer personalized support for individuals with sensory impairments (Brotosaputro et al., 2024). These advancements not only enhance independence but also promote social participation. Moreover, the use of Artificial Intelligence (AI) and Virtual Reality (VR) technologies has shown great promise in advancing inclusive education, particularly for students with disabilities (Yenduri et al., 2023). AI-driven adaptive systems dynamically tailor learning experiences to individual needs, while VR provides immersive, multi-sensory environments that foster experiential learning (Rane et al., 2023). However, challenges remain, including high costs, technical barriers, limited teacher readiness, and ethical concerns such as privacy and algorithmic bias (Regan & Jesse, 2019). Further empirical research is essential to explore the long-term impacts of AI and VR and to advocate for equitable access to these technologies in underserved educational settings (Mittal et al., 2024). Research should also focus on how these technologies can be adapted for different cultural contexts and socioeconomic realities in LMICs to ensure that innovations do not inadvertently widen existing disparities.

Telerehabilitation—the delivery of rehabilitation services via telecommunications technology—has gained prominence, especially in low- and middle-income countries (LMICs), due to its potential to overcome geographical barriers and enhance access to care. In LMICs, access to medical and rehabilitation services is often limited due to factors such as a lack of expertise, geographical challenges, and socio-cultural issues. Telerehabilitation offers a practical solution to circumvent these barriers by providing remote access to necessary services (Mohamad & Defi, 2023). Telerehabilitation also facilitates the continuation of care during emergencies, such as natural disasters or pandemics, which disproportionately impact LMICs.

However, the successful implementation of telerehabilitation in these regions faces several challenges. Limited internet access, low digital literacy, and socioeconomic disparities can hinder the equitable adoption of telerehabilitation services. For example, in Brazil, despite a significant number of internet users, a large portion of the population, particularly among the poorest, lacks adequate internet access, making it difficult to implement telerehabilitation effectively (Fernandes & Saragiotto, 2021). Additionally, low levels of digital literacy among both healthcare providers and patients can impede the adoption of these technologies. Training and education are essential to ensure the effective use of telehealth technologies to improve the sustainability of telerehabilitation, governments and international organizations need to prioritize the expansion of digital infrastructure and digital literacy programs.

Despite these challenges, there have been successful implementations of telerehabilitation in LMICs. During the COVID-19 pandemic, for instance, telerehabilitation initiatives were introduced in Bangladesh to serve both Rohingya and host communities, marking a novel approach in the region (Ahmed & Ali, 2021). Nevertheless, for telerehabilitation to be sustainable and effective, addressing infrastructural barriers and ensuring digital literacy will be key to its success. By overcoming these challenges, telerehabilitation can significantly enhance disability inclusion efforts in LMICs, improving the quality of life for individuals with disabilities.

7.2.3 Data-Driven Inclusion

Big data analytics is being leveraged to map disability demographics and identify service gaps. This data-driven approach informs policymakers and service providers, facilitating evidence-based interventions (McPherson et al., 2017). By integrating data across sectors, countries can tailor interventions to meet specific needs and maximize their impact on disability inclusion (Saran et al., 2020). This approach also facilitates better tracking of progress toward achieving SDGs related to disability inclusion, allowing for more targeted interventions and resource allocation.

Figure 7.1 illustrates the key technological advancements that have significantly contributed to improving disability inclusion in low- and middle-income countries (LMICs).

7.2.4 Social Inclusion Interventions in LMICs

Recent systematic reviews have shown that interventions targeting social inclusion outcomes for people with disabilities in LMICs have produced significant positive effects.

A review of interventions across 16 countries highlighted the positive impact of efforts to enhance social and communication skills, provide personal assistance, and strengthen relationships between individuals with disabilities and their families and communities. These initiatives demonstrated significant improvements in fostering social inclusion outcomes, particularly in building skills, improving relationships, and promoting broader inclusion (Saran et al., 2023). These interventions have also

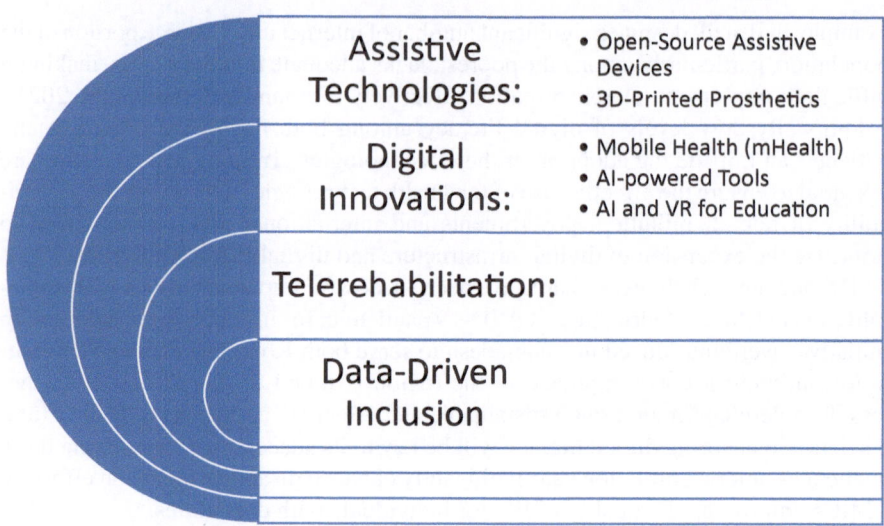

Fig. 7.1 Technological innovations advancing disability inclusion

helped reduce isolation, increase community engagement, and improve mental health among people with disabilities.

Importantly, these interventions primarily addressed individual-level barriers, such as social and communication skills, rather than systemic factors contributing to exclusion, such as stigma and inadequate infrastructure. The evidence highlights a need for interventions that not only target personal skills but also work to reduce societal stigma and strengthen legislative, infrastructural, and institutional support for inclusion.

7.3   Access to Rehabilitation Services in LMICs

A recent systematic review examining access to rehabilitation services for people with disabilities in LMICs further emphasizes the need for improvement in service delivery. The findings revealed that access to rehabilitation services, including the use of assistive devices, specialist health services, and adherence to treatment, was highly variable and generally inadequate. While some studies addressed specific impairments such as vision, hearing, physical, and mental health disabilities, there was no clear pattern regarding access based on equity measures such as age, socioeconomic status, or locality (Bright et al., 2018). This variability highlights the pressing need for equitable distribution of resources and the development of inclusive rehabilitation systems.

The study concluded that access to rehabilitation services remains insufficient in many LMICs, with significant gaps in both availability and coverage. A key limitation identified was the lack of standardized metrics and consistent measurements across studies, which made it difficult to assess the true population-level need for these services. The review called for better data collection and clinical assessments to evaluate the extent of the rehabilitation gap, and for more comprehensive studies to understand the broader needs of people with disabilities. This highlights the importance of addressing systemic barriers, including infrastructure, policy, and societal stigma, alongside efforts to improve individual skills and access to services.

7.4 Community Support for Persons with Disabilities

A scoping review of community support for persons with disabilities in LMICs highlights critical gaps and barriers in access to support services. The review found that while formal and informal strategies exist across the life course and different life domains, the evidence on their effectiveness and coverage is still limited. This lack of evidence is compounded by the absence of clear models for evaluating interventions and strategies that could provide more effective community support (Hunt et al., 2022).

The review also emphasized the role of community-based rehabilitation (CBR) and Organizations of Persons with Disabilities (OPDs) in the provision and development of community support services. However, the review pointed out that the contributions of these organizations, while important, need to be more clearly articulated in the context of community support. Moreover, the study identified a need for robust theory of change models that could evaluate the different aspects of complex interventions and guide more effective community support practices in LMICs. These findings underline the need for tailored community support models that take into account local customs, values, and available resources.

The barriers to providing community support were also evident, including limited resources, societal stigma, and a lack of infrastructure. These findings reinforce the need for integrated, inclusive policies that ensure equal access to community living for persons with disabilities across LMICs.

7.5 Innovative Care Models

7.5.1 Community-Based Rehabilitation (CBR)

CBR programs remain a cornerstone for disability inclusion in LMICs. Recent adaptations integrate technology and interdisciplinary approaches, enhancing their effectiveness. For example, community health workers equipped with mobile apps can deliver targeted interventions and monitor progress (AlHeresh et al., 2019). Furthermore, these programs have the potential to be scaled to rural and underserved areas where traditional services may not reach.

7.5.2   Family-Centered Care (FCC)

Family involvement has been recognized as a critical factor in achieving positive outcomes. FCC models emphasize collaborative goal setting and culturally sensitive practices, aligning care with patient preferences and family dynamics (Gafni-Lachter, 2015). FCC also promotes better family understanding of the needs of individuals with disabilities, helping families become strong advocates for their loved ones.

7.5.3   Inclusive Education

Innovative educational programs that incorporate assistive technologies and flexible curricula are transforming learning environments. These models address barriers faced by children with disabilities, fostering inclusivity and academic success (Gaad, 2010; Khochen-Bagshaw, 2020). Inclusive education also emphasizes teacher training and the importance of creating supportive learning environments that can accommodate a wide range of disabilities.

7.6   Policy Interventions

7.6.1   Legal Frameworks

Many LMICs have adopted policies aligned with the United Nations Convention on the Rights of Persons with Disabilities (UN CRPD). These frameworks advocate for accessible infrastructure, employment opportunities, and anti-discrimination measures (World Bank, 2024).

7.6.2   Multisectoral Collaboration

Effective disability inclusion requires coordinated efforts across sectors, including healthcare, education, and labor. Public-private partnerships have demonstrated success in scaling innovative solutions and enhancing sustainability (UNICEF, 2024).

These partnerships are crucial for ensuring that inclusive policies are not only developed but also implemented effectively.

7.6.3 Financial Incentives

Subsidies and funding programs support the development and dissemination of assistive technologies and inclusive services. For instance, microfinance initiatives empower individuals with disabilities to establish small businesses, fostering economic independence (Sarker & Khan, 2024). Financial incentives also encourage private sector involvement in the development of affordable technologies and services.

7.7 Research Agenda

Despite the progress, significant gaps remain. This chapter proposes the following research priorities:

- **Technological Equity**: Investigate strategies to reduce the digital divide, ensuring equal access to assistive technologies.
- **Inclusive Policy Implementation**: Assess the effectiveness of existing policies and identify barriers to their implementation.
- **Longitudinal Studies**: Conduct studies to evaluate the long-term impact of innovative care models on disability inclusion.
- **Cultural Contexts**: Explore culturally sensitive approaches to reduce stigma and promote inclusion.
- **Capacity Building**: Develop frameworks for training local professionals in delivering disability-inclusive services.

7.8 Conclusion

The integration of technological innovations, inclusive care models, and robust policies marks a transformative era for disability research and practice in LMICs. By addressing existing gaps and embracing emerging opportunities, stakeholders can pave the way for a more inclusive future. This chapter underscores the need for continued collaboration, innovation, and research to advance disability inclusion globally.

References

Ahmed, R., & Ali, F. (2021). Developing telerehabilitation in low-income countries during COVID-19: Commencement and acceptability of telerehabilitation in Rohingya and host community people. In S. Siuly, H. Wang, L. Chen, Y. Guo, & C. Xing (Eds.), *Health information science* (Vol. 13079). Springer. https://doi.org/10.1007/978-3-030-90885-0_3

AlHeresh, R., Griffin, M., & Li, J. (2019). Community-based rehabilitation (CBR) in low-and middle-income countries: A systematic review of strategies and interventions. *The American Journal of Occupational Therapy, 73*(4_Supplement_1). https://doi.org/10.5014/ajot.2019.73S1-PO4007

Anawade, P. A., Sharma, D., & Gahane, S. (2024). A comprehensive review on exploring the impact of telemedicine on healthcare accessibility. *Cureus, 16*(3), e55996. https://doi.org/10.7759/cureus.55996

Bright, T., Wallace, S., & Kuper, H. (2018). A systematic review of access to rehabilitation for people with disabilities in low- and middle-income countries. *International Journal of Environmental Research and Public Health, 15*(10), 2165. https://doi.org/10.3390/ijerph15102165

Brotosaputro, G., Supriyadi, A., & Jones, M. (2024). AI-powered assistive technologies for improved accessibility. *International Transactions on Artificial Intelligence (ITALIC), 3*(1), 76–84. https://doi.org/10.33050/italic.v3i1.645

Chalkiadakis, A., Seremetaki, A., Kanellou, A., Kallishi, M., Morfopoulou, A., Moraitaki, M., & Mastrokoukou, S. (2024). Impact of artificial intelligence and virtual reality on educational inclusion: A systematic review of technologies supporting students with disabilities. *Education Sciences, 14*(11), 1223. https://doi.org/10.3390/educsci14111223

Fernandes, L. G., & Saragiotto, B. T. (2021). To what extent can telerehabilitation help patients in low- and middle-income countries? *Brazilian Journal of Physical Therapy, 25*(5), 481–483. https://doi.org/10.1016/j.bjpt.2020.11.004

Gaad, E. (2010). *Inclusive education in the Middle East*. Routledge.

Gafni-Lachter, L. R. (2015). *Better together: Advancing family centered care* (Doctoral dissertation, Boston University).

Goshe, M. T., & Kassegne, S. K. (2022). *Three-dimensional (3d) printing: Cost-effective solution for increased access to prosthesis of lower extremity*. Case of Ethiopia.

Haleem, A., Javaid, M., Singh, R. P., & Suman, R. (2021). Telemedicine for healthcare: Capabilities, features, barriers, and applications. *Sensors International, 2*, 100117. https://doi.org/10.1016/j.sintl.2021.100117

Hunt, X., Bradshaw, M., Vogel, S. L., Encalada, A. V., Eksteen, S., Schneider, M., Chunga, K., & Swartz, L. (2022). Community support for persons with disabilities in low- and middle-income countries: A scoping review. *International Journal of Environmental Research and Public Health, 19*(14), 8269. https://doi.org/10.3390/ijerph19148269

Khochen-Bagshaw, M. (2020). Inclusive education development and challenges: Insights into the Middle East and North Africa region. *Prospects, 49*(3), 153–167.

McPherson, A., Durham, J., Richards, N., Gouda, H., Rampatige, R., & Whittaker, M. (2017). Strengthening health information systems for disability-related rehabilitation in LMICs. *Health Policy and Planning, 32*(3), 384–394. https://doi.org/10.1093/heapol/czw140

Mittal, S., Vashist, S., & Chaudhary, K. (2024). Equitable education and sustainable learning: A literary exploration of integration of artificial intelligence in education for SDGs advancement. In T. Singh, S. Dutta, S. Vyas, & Á. Rocha (Eds.), *Explainable AI for education: Recent trends and challenges* (Vol. 19). Information Systems Engineering and Management. Springer. https://doi.org/10.1007/978-3-031-72410-7_6

Rane, N., Choudhary, S., & Rane, J. (2023). *Education 4.0 and 5.0: Integrating artificial intelligence (AI) for personalized and adaptive learning*.

Regan, P. M., & Jesse, J. (2019). Ethical challenges of edtech, big data and personalized learning: Twenty-first century student sorting and tracking. *Ethics and Information Technology, 21*, 167–179.

Sabrina Mohamad, I., & Ruslina Defi, I. (2023). Telerehabilitation in low- and middle-income countries. *IntechOpen*. https://doi.org/10.5772/intechopen.107449

Saran, A., Hunt, X., White, H., & Kuper, H. (2023). Effectiveness of interventions for improving social inclusion outcomes for people with disabilities in low- and middle-income countries: A systematic review. *Campbell Systematic Reviews, 19*, e1316. https://doi.org/10.1002/cl2.1316

Saran, A., White, H., & Kuper, H. (2020). Evidence and gap map of studies assessing the effectiveness of interventions for people with disabilities in low-and middle-income countries. *Campbell Systematic Reviews, 16*(1), e1070. https://doi.org/10.1002/cl2.1070

Sarker, D., & Khan, M. A. (2024). Microfinance and economic and social empowerment of people with disabilities: Lessons from Bangladesh. *Development Policy Review, 42*, e12799. https://doi.org/10.1111/dpr.12799

UNICEF. (2024). *An inclusive world starts with me, with you, with all of us*. https://www.unicef.org/media/134511/file/An%20inclusive%20world,%20starts%20with%20me,%20with%20you,%20with%20all%20of%20us.pdf

UNRIC. (2024, December 30). *Building an accessible future for all: AI and the inclusion of persons with disabilities*. United Nations Regional Information Centre for Western Europe. https://unric.org/en/building-an-accessible-future-for-all-ai-and-the-inclusion-of-persons-with-disabilities/?utm_source=chatgpt.com

World Bank. (2024). *Disability inclusion and the United Nations Convention on the Rights of Persons with Disabilities (UN CRPD)*. World Bank Group.

Yenduri, G., Kaluri, R., Rajput, D. S., Lakshmana, K., Gadekallu, T. R., Mahmud, M., & Brown, D. J. (2023). From assistive technologies to metaverse—Technologies in inclusive higher education for students with specific learning difficulties: A review. *IEEE Access, 11*, 64907–64927.